I0711082

Welcome to ***"Type 2 Diabetes Cookbook After 50: 110+ Recipes to Help Control Blood Sugar and Boost Wellbeing."*** Whether you've recently been diagnosed with type 2 diabetes or have been managing it for some time, this cookbook is designed to make your culinary journey both enjoyable and healthful. Living with diabetes doesn't mean you have to sacrifice flavor or variety in your meals. In fact, with the right recipes, you can savor delicious dishes while keeping your blood sugar levels in check and supporting your overall wellbeing.

As we age, our nutritional needs change, and managing type 2 diabetes adds another layer of consideration to our diets. This book is tailored specifically for those over 50, recognizing the unique challenges and opportunities that come with this stage of life. The recipes here are crafted to provide balanced nutrition, enhance energy levels, and support heart health, all while being mindful of blood sugar management.

In this book, you'll find a wide range of recipes that cater to different tastes and preferences. From hearty breakfasts that kickstart your day to satisfying dinners that wrap it up, each recipe is designed with care. We've also included snacks and desserts that allow you to indulge without compromising your health goals.

Our recipes focus on using whole, minimally processed ingredients that are rich in essential nutrients. You'll discover new ways to incorporate fiber, lean proteins, healthy fats, and low-glycemic carbohydrates into your meals. Each recipe includes nutritional information to help you make informed choices and maintain balanced blood sugar levels.

Managing type 2 diabetes is about more than just food. It's about adopting a holistic approach to your health. This cookbook encourages you to embrace a lifestyle that includes regular physical activity, adequate hydration, and mindfulness practices. Together, these elements can significantly improve your quality of life and help you thrive.

As you embark on this culinary journey, we hope you find joy and satisfaction in preparing and savoring these recipes. Let this book be your companion in achieving better health and wellbeing, one delicious meal at a time.

Here's to a healthier, happier you!

Happy cooking,

1. Greek Yogurt with Berries and Nuts

Instructions

1. Spoon the Greek yogurt into a bowl.

2. Top the yogurt with the mixed berries.

3. Sprinkle the chopped nuts over the top.

4. If desired, drizzle the honey over the top.

This recipe is a great option for men with type 2 diabetes for a few reasons:

1. Greek yogurt is high in protein and low in carbs, which can help manage blood sugar levels.

2. Berries are a source of fiber, vitamins, and antioxidants, and have a low glycemic index, meaning they won't spike blood sugar levels.

3. Nuts provide healthy fats, protein, and fiber, which can also help with blood sugar control.

4. The honey is optional, as it does contain some carbs, but a small amount can add a touch of sweetness.

This simple, nutrient•dense snack or breakfast can be a delicious and diabetes•friendly choice. Enjoy!

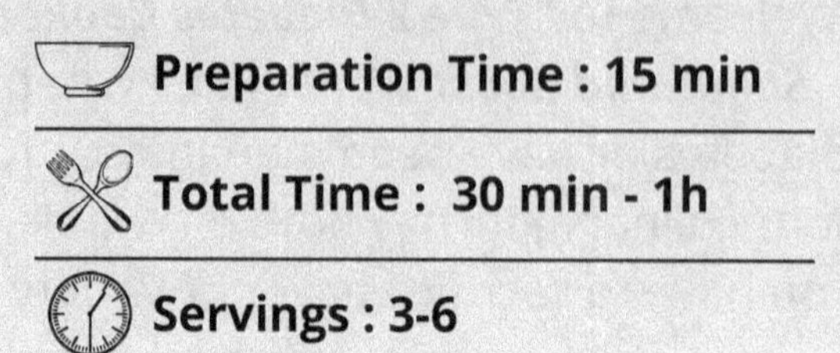

Ingredients

• 1 cup plain Greek yogurt
• 1/2 cup mixed berries (such as blueberries, raspberries, and/or blackberries)
• 2 tablespoons chopped nuts (such as almonds, walnuts, or pecans)
• 1 teaspoon honey (optional)

Instructions

1. Crack the eggs into a small bowl and beat them lightly with the milk or water. Season with a pinch of salt and pepper.

2. Heat a small non•stick skillet over medium heat and melt the butter or heat the oil.

3. Add the mushrooms and sauté for 2•3 minutes until softened.

4. Add the spinach leaves and cook for 1 minute, stirring, until the spinach is wilted.

5. Pour the egg mixture into the skillet. As the eggs start to set around the edges, use a spatula to gently push cooked egg towards the center, tilting the pan to allow uncooked egg to flow to the edges.

6. When the eggs are mostly set but still a bit runny on top, sprinkle the grated cheese (if using) over half of the omelet.

7. Fold the plain half of the omelet over the cheese half.

8. Slide the folded omelet onto a plate and serve immediately.

Enjoy your delicious vegetable•packed omelet!

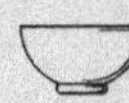 **Preparation Time : 15 min**

 **Total Time : 30 min - 1h**

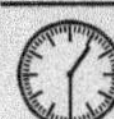 **Servings : 3-6**

Ingredients

- 3 eggs
- 2 tbsp milk or water
- 1 tsp butter or oil
- 1/2 cup sliced mushrooms
- 1 cup fresh spinach leaves
- 1 tbsp grated cheese (optional)
- Salt and pepper to taste

Instructions

1. In a medium bowl, whisk together the chia seeds, almond milk, vanilla extract, and cinnamon until well combined.

2. If using a sweetener, add the erythritol or stevia and stir until dissolved.

3. Cover the bowl and refrigerate for at least 4 hours, or overnight.

4. When ready to serve, give the pudding a good stir. The chia seeds will have absorbed the liquid and created a thick, pudding•like consistency.

5. Divide the chia pudding between two bowls or jars. Top each serving with 2 tablespoons of fresh berries.

Nutritional Info (per serving):
• Calories: 160
• Total Carbs: 13g
• Fiber: 9g
• Net Carbs: 4g
• Protein: 5g
• Fat: 9g

This chia pudding is high in fiber, low in net carbs, and contains healthy fats from the chia seeds and almond milk. The berries provide antioxidants and additional fiber. It's a great make•ahead breakfast or snack option for men managing type 2 diabetes.

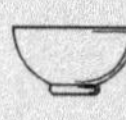 **Preparation Time : 15 min**

 **Total Time : 30 min - 1h**

 **Servings : 3-6**

Ingredients

• 1/4 cup chia seeds
• 1 cup unsweetened almond milk (or other low•sugar milk alternative)
• 1 tsp vanilla extract
• 1/2 tsp ground cinnamon
• 1•2 tbsp granulated erythritol or stevia (optional, to taste)
• 1/4 cup fresh berries (such as raspberries, blueberries or blackberries)

Instructions

1. Toast the whole grain bread slices until lightly golden brown.

2. In a small bowl, mash the avocado with a fork. Stir in the lemon juice, garlic powder, cumin, and a pinch of salt and pepper.

3. Spread the mashed avocado evenly over the toasted bread slices.

4. If using, sprinkle the crumbled feta cheese and chopped fresh herbs over the top.

Nutritional Info (per serving):
• Calories: 220
• Total Carbs: 22g
• Fiber: 8g
• Net Carbs: 14g
• Protein: 6g
• Fat: 13g

This avocado toast is a great option for men managing type 2 diabetes. The whole grain bread provides complex carbs and fiber, while the avocado adds healthy monounsaturated fats and fiber. The optional feta cheese provides a

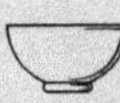 **Preparation Time : 15 min**

 **Total Time : 30 min - 1h**

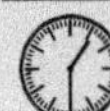 **Servings : 3-6**

Ingredients

• 2 slices of whole grain or sprouted bread
• 1 medium ripe avocado, mashed
• 1 tbsp fresh lemon juice
• 1/4 tsp garlic powder
• 1/4 tsp ground cumin
• Salt and pepper to taste
• 1 tbsp crumbled feta cheese (optional)
• 1 tbsp chopped fresh cilantro or parsley (optional)

Instructions

1. Add all the ingredients to a high•speed blender. Blend on high speed until smooth and creamy, about 1 minute.

2. Taste and adjust sweetener (erythritol or stevia) if desired. The blueberries provide natural sweetness, so you may not need any additional sweetener.

3. Pour the smoothie into a glass and enjoy immediately.

Nutritional Info (per serving):
• Calories: 150
• Total Carbs: 15g
• Fiber: 7g
• Net Carbs: 8g
• Protein: 5g
• Fat: 8g

This smoothie is an excellent choice for men managing type 2 diabetes. It's high in fiber, low in net carbs, and provides a good source of healthy fats from the almond milk and flaxseeds. The kale adds important vitamins, minerals, and antioxidants, while the blueberries provide natural sweetness and additional fiber.

The optional sweetener can be adjusted to your taste preferences. This smoothie makes a nutritious and satisfying breakfast or snack.

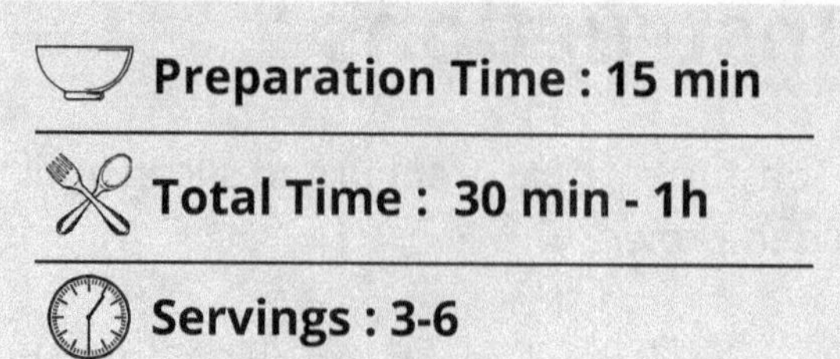

Ingredients

• 1 cup unsweetened almond milk
• 1 cup packed kale leaves, stems removed
• 1/2 cup frozen blueberries
• 1 tbsp ground flaxseeds
• 1 tsp vanilla extract
• 1•2 tsp granulated erythritol or stevia (optional, to taste)

Instructions

1. Heat the olive oil in a large non•stick skillet over medium heat. Add the diced bell pepper and onion. Sauté for 3•4 minutes until softened.

2. Add the sliced mushrooms and continue cooking for 2•3 minutes.

3. Crumble the tofu into the skillet and stir to combine with the vegetables.

4. Add the soy sauce/tamari, turmeric, garlic powder, cumin, and a pinch of salt and pepper. Stir well to coat the tofu and vegetables.

5. Add the baby spinach leaves and cook for 1•2 minutes, stirring frequently, until the spinach is wilted.

6. Remove from heat and serve the scrambled tofu and veggie mixture warm.

Nutritional Info (per serving):
• Calories: 180
• Total Carbs: 10g
• Fiber: 4g
• Net Carbs: 6g
• Protein: 16g
• Fat: 10g

This scrambled tofu dish is high in protein, low in net carbs, and packed with fiber•rich vegetables. The turmeric and cumin add great flavor. It's a nutritious and satisfying meal for men managing type 2 diabetes.

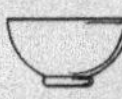 **Preparation Time : 15 min**

 **Total Time : 30 min - 1h**

 **Servings : 3-6**

Ingredients

• 1 block (14 oz) firm or extra•firm tofu, drained and crumbled
• 1 tbsp olive oil
• 1/2 cup diced bell pepper
• 1/2 cup diced onion
• 1 cup sliced mushrooms
• 2 cups baby spinach leaves
• 2 tbsp low•sodium soy sauce or tamari
• 1 tsp ground turmeric
• 1/2 tsp garlic powder
• 1/4 tsp ground cumin
• Salt and pepper to taste

7. Steel•Cut Oats with Cinnamon and Walnuts

Instructions

1. In a medium saucepan, bring the almond milk to a boil over medium•high heat.

2. Once boiling, stir in the steel•cut oats and reduce heat to low. Simmer, stirring occasionally, for 20•25 minutes, until the oats are tender and have reached your desired consistency.

3. Remove from heat and stir in the ground cinnamon. If using a sweetener, add the erythritol or stevia and stir until dissolved.

4. Transfer the cooked oatmeal to bowls and top each serving with 1 tablespoon of chopped walnuts.

5. For extra fiber, you can also sprinkle 1 tablespoon of ground flaxseeds over the top (optional).

Nutritional Info (per serving):
• Calories: 250
• Total Carbs: 30g
• Fiber: 6g
• Net Carbs: 24g
• Protein: 8g
• Fat: 10g

This steel•cut oatmeal dish is a great breakfast choice for men managing type 2 diabetes. The steel•cut oats provide complex carbs and fiber, while the walnuts add healthy fats and the cinnamon provides antioxidants. The optional sweetener can be adjusted to your taste preferences.

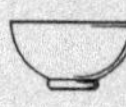 **Preparation Time : 15 min**

 **Total Time : 30 min - 1h**

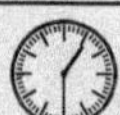 **Servings : 3-6**

Ingredients

• 1 cup steel•cut oats
• 3 cups unsweetened almond milk (or low•fat dairy milk)
• 1/4 tsp ground cinnamon
• 1 tbsp chopped walnuts
• 1•2 tsp granulated erythritol or stevia (optional)
• 1 tbsp ground flaxseeds (optional)

Instructions

1. Toast the whole grain English muffin until lightly golden brown.

2. Spread 2 tablespoons of natural peanut butter evenly over the toasted muffin halves.

3. If desired, sprinkle the chia seeds and ground flaxseeds over the peanut butter for added fiber and nutrients.

Nutritional Info (per serving):
• Calories: 250
• Total Carbs: 25g
• Fiber: 6g
• Net Carbs: 19g
• Protein: 12g
• Fat: 12g

This whole grain English muffin with peanut butter is a great breakfast or snack option for men managing type 2 diabetes. The whole grains provide complex carbs and fiber, while the peanut butter adds protein and healthy fats to help keep blood sugar levels stable.

The optional chia and flaxseeds further boost the fiber and nutrient content of this snack. Be sure to choose a natural peanut butter with no added sugars.

This is a simple, satisfying, and diabetes•friendly option that can be enjoyed on its own or paired with a piece of fruit for a more complete meal.

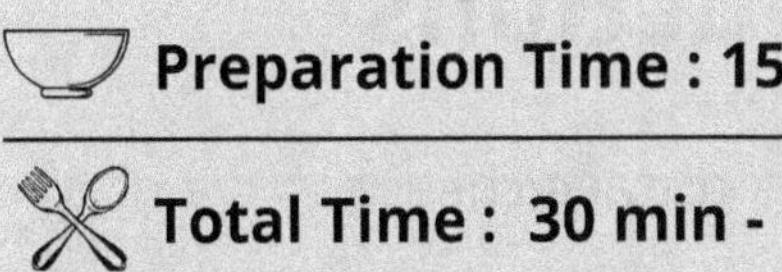

Preparation Time : 15 min

Total Time : 30 min - 1h

Servings : 3-6

Ingredients

• 1 whole grain English muffin
• 2 tbsp natural peanut butter (no added sugar)
• 1 tsp chia seeds (optional)
• 1 tsp ground flaxseeds (optional)

Instructions

1. Scoop the cottage cheese into a bowl or container.

2. Top the cottage cheese with the mixed fresh berries.

3. If desired, sprinkle the chopped nuts over the top.

4. Drizzle with a small amount of honey or maple syrup, if using. Start with 1 tsp and add more to taste.

Nutritional Info (per serving):
• Calories: 200
• Total Carbs: 15g
• Fiber: 4g
• Net Carbs: 11g
• Protein: 20g
• Fat: 7g

This cottage cheese and fruit combination is an excellent snack or light meal for men managing type 2 diabetes. The cottage cheese provides a good source of protein, while the fresh berries add fiber, vitamins, and natural sweetness.

The optional nuts add healthy fats and extra crunch. The small amount of honey or maple syrup can be adjusted to your taste preferences, or omitted entirely if you prefer a less sweet option.

This is a simple, nutrient•dense, and diabetes•friendly snack that can be enjoyed any time of day.

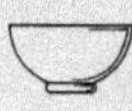 **Preparation Time : 15 min**

 **Total Time : 30 min - 1h**

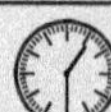 **Servings : 3-6**

Ingredients

• 1 cup low•fat or non•fat cottage cheese
• 1 cup mixed fresh berries (such as blueberries, raspberries, blackberries)
• 1 tbsp chopped walnuts or sliced almonds (optional)
• 1 tsp honey or maple syrup (optional)

Instructions

1. In a bowl, combine the cooked and cooled quinoa with the unsweetened almond milk.

2. Top the quinoa mixture with the fresh berries.

3. Sprinkle the chopped nuts and ground cinnamon over the top.

4. If desired, add 1•2 tsp of granulated erythritol or stevia to sweeten the dish slightly.

Nutritional Info (per serving):
• Calories: 250
• Total Carbs: 30g
• Fiber: 7g
• Net Carbs: 23g
• Protein: 8g
• Fat: 12g

This quinoa breakfast bowl is a great option for men managing type 2 diabetes. Quinoa is a whole grain that is high in fiber and protein, helping to keep blood sugar levels stable. The berries provide natural sweetness, antioxidants, and additional fiber.

The nuts add healthy fats and crunch, while the cinnamon provides antioxidants and may help regulate blood sugar levels. The optional sweetener can be adjusted to your taste preferences.

This breakfast bowl is a nutritious and satisfying way to start the day. It can be prepared ahead of time for a quick and easy morning meal.

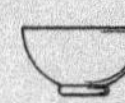 **Preparation Time : 15 min**

 **Total Time : 30 min - 1h**

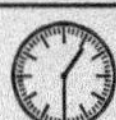 **Servings : 3-6**

Ingredients

• 1/2 cup cooked quinoa, cooled
• 1/2 cup unsweetened almond milk
• 1/2 cup fresh berries (such as blueberries, raspberries, or blackberries)
• 1 tbsp chopped walnuts or sliced almonds
• 1 tsp ground cinnamon
• 1•2 tsp granulated erythritol or stevia (optional)

Instructions

1. In a large salad bowl, combine the mixed greens, cherry tomatoes, and sliced cucumber.

2. Top the salad with the grilled chicken slices and crumbled feta cheese.

3. In a small bowl, whisk together the olive oil, balsamic vinegar, Dijon mustard, and lemon juice to make the dressing.

4. Drizzle the olive oil dressing over the salad and toss gently to coat.

5. Season with salt and pepper to taste.

Nutritional Info (per serving):
• Calories: 300
• Total Carbs: 12g
• Fiber: 4g
• Net Carbs: 8g
• Protein: 32g
• Fat: 16g

This grilled chicken salad is an excellent option for men managing type 2 diabetes. The mixed greens provide fiber and nutrients, while the grilled chicken adds lean protein. The healthy fats from the olive oil and feta cheese help to slow the absorption of carbohydrates.

The simple olive oil and balsamic vinegar dressing is low in added sugars, making it a diabetes•friendly choice. This salad is filling, nutritious, and can be easily customized with your favorite greens and toppings.

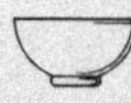 Preparation Time : 15 min

 Total Time : 30 min - 1h

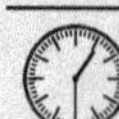 Servings : 3-6

Ingredients

• 4 oz grilled chicken breast, sliced
• 2 cups mixed greens (such as spinach, arugula, kale)
• 1/2 cup cherry tomatoes, halved
• 1/4 cup sliced cucumber
• 2 tbsp crumbled feta cheese
• 1 tbsp olive oil
• 1 tbsp balsamic vinegar
• 1 tsp Dijon mustard
• 1 tsp lemon juice
• Salt and pepper to taste

12. Lentil Soup with Vegetables

Instructions

1. In a large pot, bring the broth to a boil over high heat. Add the rinsed lentils, reduce heat to medium•low, and simmer for 15•20 minutes, until lentils are tender.

2. Meanwhile, in a separate skillet, heat the olive oil over medium heat. Add the diced onion, carrots, and celery. Sauté for 5•7 minutes until softened.

3. Add the minced garlic, cumin, oregano, and red pepper flakes (if using). Cook for 1 minute until fragrant.

4. Transfer the sautéed vegetables to the pot with the cooked lentils. Add the can of diced tomatoes (with juices) and the chopped kale or spinach.

5. Simmer the soup for an additional 10 minutes, allowing the flavors to meld and the greens to wilt.

6. Season with salt and pepper to taste.

Nutritional Info (per serving):
• Calories: 250
• Total Carbs: 35g
• Fiber: 12g
• Net Carbs: 23g
• Protein: 15g
• Fat: 6g

This lentil soup is packed with fiber, protein, and nutrients, making it an excellent choice for men managing type 2 diabetes. The vegetables and spices add great flavor without added sugars. Enjoy this hearty and satisfying soup!

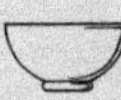 **Preparation Time : 15 min**

 **Total Time : 30 min - 1h**

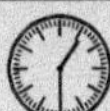 **Servings : 3-6**

Ingredients

• 1 cup dry brown or green lentils, rinsed
• 4 cups low•sodium vegetable or chicken broth
• 1 tbsp olive oil
• 1 medium onion, diced
• 2 carrots, peeled and diced
• 2 celery stalks, diced
• 3 garlic cloves, minced
• 1 tsp ground cumin
• 1 tsp dried oregano
• 1/4 tsp red pepper flakes (optional)
• 1 (14.5 oz) can diced tomatoes
• 2 cups chopped kale or spinach
• Salt and pepper to taste

Instructions

1. Lay the whole wheat tortilla flat on a clean surface.

2. Spread the hummus evenly over the center of the tortilla.

3. Layer the sliced turkey breast, avocado slices, and shredded lettuce on top of the hummus.

4. Drizzle the olive oil and balsamic vinegar over the filling.

5. Season with a pinch of salt and pepper.

6. Fold the bottom of the tortilla up over the filling, then fold in the sides and continue rolling tightly into a wrap.

7. Cut the wrap in half diagonally and serve.

Nutritional Info (per serving):
• Calories: 320
• Total Carbs: 25g
• Fiber: 7g
• Net Carbs: 18g
• Protein: 22g
• Fat: 16g

This turkey and avocado wrap is a great option for men managing type 2 diabetes. The whole wheat tortilla provides complex carbs and fiber, while the turkey and avocado offer a balance of protein and healthy fats.

The hummus adds extra fiber and creaminess, and the olive oil and balsamic vinegar dressing provides flavor without added sugars. This wrap is portable, satisfying, and packed with nutrients to help keep blood sugar levels stable.

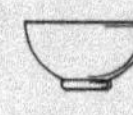 **Preparation Time : 15 min**

 **Total Time : 30 min - 1h**

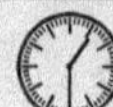 **Servings : 3-6**

Ingredients

• 1 whole wheat tortilla (8•10 inches)
• 3 oz sliced turkey breast
• 1/2 avocado, sliced
• 1/4 cup shredded lettuce
• 1 tbsp hummus
• 1 tsp olive oil
• 1 tsp balsamic vinegar
• Salt and pepper to taste

Instructions

1. In a large bowl, combine the cooked and cooled quinoa, rinsed black beans, diced cucumber, red bell pepper, red onion, and chopped cilantro.

2. In a small bowl, whisk together the olive oil, lime juice, cumin, and chili powder. Season with a pinch of salt and pepper.

3. Pour the dressing over the quinoa and bean salad and toss gently to coat.

4. Refrigerate the salad for at least 30 minutes to allow the flavors to meld.

5. Serve chilled or at room temperature.

Nutritional Info (per serving):
• Calories: 220
• Total Carbs: 28g
• Fiber: 8g
• Net Carbs: 20g
• Protein: 8g
• Fat: 9g

This quinoa and black bean salad is an excellent choice for men managing type 2 diabetes. The combination of quinoa, a high•fiber whole grain, and black beans, a good source of protein and fiber, helps to keep blood sugar levels stable.

The fresh vegetables, herbs, and simple dressing add flavor and nutrients without added sugars. This salad can be enjoyed as a main dish or a side, and it's easy to prepare in advance for a quick and healthy meal.

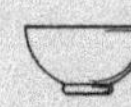 **Preparation Time : 15 min**

 **Total Time : 30 min - 1h**

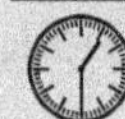 **Servings : 3-6**

Ingredients

• 1 cup cooked quinoa, cooled
• 1 (15 oz) can black beans, rinsed and drained
• 1 cup diced cucumber
• 1/2 cup diced red bell pepper
• 1/4 cup diced red onion
• 2 tbsp chopped fresh cilantro
• 2 tbsp olive oil
• 1 tbsp lime juice
• 1 tsp ground cumin
• 1/4 tsp chili powder
• Salt and pepper to taste

Instructions

1. In a large salad bowl, combine the chopped romaine lettuce, cherry tomatoes, diced cucumber, sliced red onion, and halved kalamata olives.

2. In a small bowl, whisk together the olive oil, red wine vinegar, dried oregano, Dijon mustard, and minced garlic. Season with a pinch of salt and pepper.

3. Drizzle the vinaigrette over the salad and toss gently to coat.

4. Sprinkle the crumbled feta cheese over the top of the salad.

Nutritional Info (per serving):
• Calories: 200
• Total Carbs: 10g
• Fiber: 3g
• Net Carbs: 7g
• Protein: 8g
• Fat: 16g

This Greek salad is an excellent choice for men managing type 2 diabetes. The leafy greens, vegetables, and olives provide fiber, vitamins, and antioxidants. The feta cheese adds protein and healthy fats to help slow the absorption of carbohydrates.

The simple olive oil and red wine vinegar dressing is low in added sugars, making it a diabetes•friendly option. This salad is refreshing, satisfying, and can be easily customized with your favorite Mediterranean•inspired ingredients.

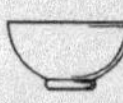 **Preparation Time : 15 min**

 **Total Time : 30 min - 1h**

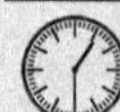 **Servings : 3-6**

Ingredients

• 6 cups chopped romaine lettuce
• 1 cup cherry tomatoes, halved
• 1/2 cup diced cucumber
• 1/4 cup sliced red onion
• 1/4 cup pitted kalamata olives, halved
• 2 oz crumbled feta cheese
• 2 tbsp olive oil
• 1 tbsp red wine vinegar
• 1 tsp dried oregano
• 1 tsp Dijon mustard
• 1 clove garlic, minced
• Salt and pepper to taste

Instructions

1. Cook the brown rice according to package instructions. Set aside.

2. In a small bowl, combine the soy sauce, rice vinegar, and sesame oil. Set aside.

3. Heat the olive oil in a large skillet or wok over high heat. Add the chicken and stir•fry for 3•4 minutes until lightly browned.

4. Add the minced garlic and grated ginger to the skillet. Stir•fry for 1 minute until fragrant.

5. Add the broccoli, mushrooms, bell pepper, and snow/snap peas. Stir•fry for 4•5 minutes until the vegetables are tender•crisp.

6. Pour the soy sauce mixture into the skillet and toss everything together to coat.

7. Serve the chicken and vegetable stir•fry over the cooked brown rice. Garnish with sliced green onions.

Nutritional Info (per serving):
• Calories: 350
• Total Carbs: 30g
• Fiber: 6g
• Net Carbs: 24g
• Protein: 35g

This chicken and vegetable stir•fry with brown rice is an excellent choice for men managing type 2 diabetes. The lean protein from the chicken, fiber•rich vegetables, and whole grain brown rice provide a balanced, nutrient•dense meal.

The simple soy sauce and rice vinegar dressing adds flavor without added sugars. This dish is easy to prepare and can be customized with your favorite stir•fry vegetables.

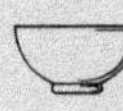 **Preparation Time : 15 min**

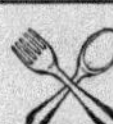 **Total Time : 30 min - 1h**

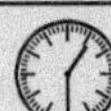 **Servings : 3-6**

Ingredients

• 1 cup cooked brown rice
• 1 lb boneless, skinless chicken breasts, cut into 1•inch pieces
• 2 tbsp low•sodium soy sauce or tamari
• 1 tbsp rice vinegar
• 1 tsp sesame oil
• 1 tbsp olive oil
• 2 cloves garlic, minced
• 1 inch piece fresh ginger, peeled and grated
• 1 cup broccoli florets
• 1 cup sliced mushrooms
• 1 red bell pepper, sliced
• 1 cup snow peas or snap peas
• 2 green onions, sliced
• Salt and pepper to taste

Instructions

1. In a medium bowl, gently mix together the drained tuna, rinsed chickpeas, diced celery, red onion, and chopped parsley.

2. In a small bowl, whisk together the olive oil, lemon juice, Dijon mustard, and honey (if using). Season with a pinch of salt and pepper.

3. Pour the lemon vinaigrette over the tuna and chickpea mixture and toss gently to coat.

4. Refrigerate the salad for at least 30 minutes to allow the flavors to meld.

5. Serve chilled or at room temperature.

Nutritional Info (per serving):
• Calories: 250
• Total Carbs: 20g
• Fiber: 6g
• Net Carbs: 14g
• Protein: 20g
• Fat: 12g

This tuna salad with chickpeas is an excellent choice for men managing type 2 diabetes. The combination of tuna, a lean protein, and chickpeas, a high•fiber legume, helps to keep blood sugar levels stable.

The lemon vinaigrette dressing is low in added sugars, providing a bright, tangy flavor without spiking blood sugar. This salad can be enjoyed on its own, over a bed of greens, or stuffed into a whole grain pita or wrap.

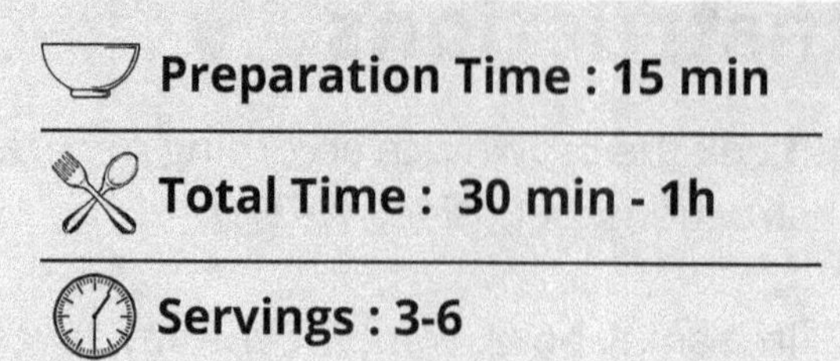

Preparation Time : 15 min

Total Time : 30 min - 1h

Servings : 3-6

Ingredients

• 1 (5 oz) can tuna, drained
• 1 (15 oz) can chickpeas, rinsed and drained
• 1/2 cup diced celery
• 1/4 cup diced red onion
• 2 tbsp chopped parsley
• 2 tbsp olive oil
• 1 tbsp lemon juice
• 1 tsp Dijon mustard
• 1 tsp honey (optional)
• Salt and pepper to taste

Instructions

1. Bring a large pot of salted water to a boil. Cook the whole grain pasta according to package instructions until al dente. Drain and set aside.

2. In a large bowl, combine the cooked pasta, basil pesto, and halved cherry tomatoes. Toss gently to coat the pasta.

3. Sprinkle the pine nuts or chopped walnuts and grated Parmesan cheese over the top.

4. Drizzle the olive oil over the pasta and season with salt and pepper to taste.

5. Serve warm or at room temperature.

Nutritional Info (per serving):
• Calories: 350
• Total Carbs: 40g
• Fiber: 8g
• Net Carbs: 32g
• Protein: 14g
• Fat: 16g

This whole grain pasta dish is a great option for men managing type 2 diabetes. The whole grain pasta provides complex carbs and fiber, while the pesto, cherry tomatoes, and nuts add healthy fats, protein, and antioxidants.

The Parmesan cheese provides a creamy, savory element without adding a significant amount of carbs. This pasta can be enjoyed as a main dish or a side, and it's easy to prepare in advance for a quick and diabetes•friendly meal.

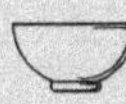 **Preparation Time : 15 min**

 **Total Time : 30 min - 1h**

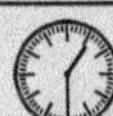 **Servings : 3-6**

Ingredients

• 8 oz whole grain pasta (such as whole wheat or chickpea pasta)
• 1/2 cup basil pesto (store•bought or homemade)
• 1 cup cherry tomatoes, halved
• 2 tbsp pine nuts or chopped walnuts
• 2 tbsp grated Parmesan cheese
• 1 tbsp olive oil
• Salt and pepper to taste

Instructions

1. Lay the whole wheat tortilla or wrap flat on a clean surface.

2. Spread the hummus evenly over the center of the tortilla.

3. Layer the mixed greens, sliced cucumber, bell pepper, and shredded carrots on top of the hummus.

4. If using, sprinkle the crumbled feta cheese over the vegetables.

5. Drizzle the olive oil and balsamic vinegar over the filling.

6. Season with a pinch of salt and pepper.

7. Fold the bottom of the tortilla up over the filling, then fold in the sides and continue rolling tightly into a wrap. Cut the wrap in half diagonally and serve.

Nutritional Info (per serving):
• Calories: 280
• Total Carbs: 35g
• Fiber: 8g
• Net Carbs: 27g
• Protein: 10g
• Fat: 12g

This hummus and veggie wrap is a great option for men managing type 2 diabetes. The whole wheat tortilla provides complex carbs and fiber, while the hummus, vegetables, and optional feta cheese offer a balance of protein, healthy fats, and additional fiber.

The olive oil and balsamic vinegar dressing adds flavor without added sugars. This wrap is portable, satisfying, and packed with nutrients to help keep blood sugar levels stable.

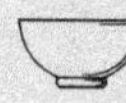 **Preparation Time : 15 min**

 **Total Time : 30 min - 1h**

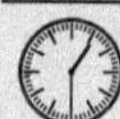 **Servings : 3-6**

Ingredients

• 1 whole wheat tortilla or wrap (8•10 inches)
• 2•3 tbsp hummus
• 1/2 cup mixed greens (such as spinach, arugula, or kale)
• 1/4 cup sliced cucumber
• 1/4 cup sliced bell pepper
• 2 tbsp shredded carrots
• 1 tbsp crumbled feta cheese (optional)
• 1 tsp olive oil
• 1 tsp balsamic vinegar
• Salt and pepper to taste

Instructions

1. Preheat oven to 375°F. Place the bell pepper halves in a baking dish and set aside.

2. In a large skillet over medium heat, cook the ground turkey, breaking it up as it cooks, until no longer pink, about 5•7 minutes.

3. Add the diced onion and minced garlic to the skillet. Cook for 2•3 minutes until the onion is translucent.

4. Stir in the cooked quinoa, diced tomatoes, oregano, cumin, and red pepper flakes (if using). Season with salt and pepper to taste.

5. Spoon the turkey and quinoa mixture evenly into the bell pepper halves.

6. Top each stuffed pepper with a sprinkle of shredded mozzarella cheese. Bake for 20•25 minutes, until the peppers are tender and the cheese is melted.

Nutritional Info (per serving):
• Calories: 300
• Total Carbs: 20g
• Fiber: 5g
• Net Carbs: 15g
• Protein: 30g

These stuffed bell peppers are a great option for men managing type 2 diabetes. The combination of lean ground turkey, quinoa, and vegetables provides a balanced, nutrient•dense meal. The fiber and protein help to keep blood sugar levels stable.

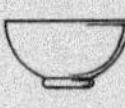
Preparation Time : 15 min

Total Time : 30 min - 1h

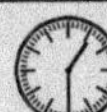
Servings : 3-6

Ingredients

• 4 medium bell peppers, halved lengthwise and seeds removed
• 1 lb ground turkey
• 1 cup cooked quinoa
• 1 small onion, diced
• 2 cloves garlic, minced
• 1 (14.5 oz) can diced tomatoes
• 1 tsp dried oregano
• 1 tsp ground cumin
• 1/4 tsp red pepper flakes (optional)
• 1/2 cup shredded mozzarella cheese
• Salt and pepper to taste

Instructions

1. Preheat oven to 400°F. Line a baking sheet with parchment paper.

2. Place the salmon fillets on one side of the prepared baking sheet. Arrange the trimmed asparagus spears on the other side.

3. In a small bowl, whisk together the olive oil, lemon juice, Dijon mustard, and dried dill. Season with a pinch of salt and pepper.

4. Drizzle the oil and lemon mixture over the salmon and asparagus, making sure to coat everything evenly.

5. Bake for 12•15 minutes, or until the salmon is cooked through and flakes easily with a fork, and the asparagus is tender•crisp. Serve the baked salmon and asparagus immediately.

Nutritional Info (per serving):
• Calories: 300
• Total Carbs: 8g
• Fiber: 4g
• Net Carbs: 4g
• Protein: 35g
• Fat: 16g

This baked salmon and asparagus dish is an excellent choice for men managing type 2 diabetes. Salmon is a great source of lean protein and healthy omega•3 fatty acids, while asparagus provides fiber, vitamins, and minerals.

The simple lemon•Dijon dressing adds flavor without added sugars. This meal is easy to prepare, nutrient•dense, and can be enjoyed as a complete, diabetes•friendly dinner.

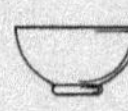 **Preparation Time : 15 min**

 **Total Time : 30 min - 1h**

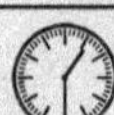 **Servings : 3-6**

Ingredients

• 4 (4 oz) salmon fillets
• 1 lb asparagus, trimmed
• 2 tbsp olive oil
• 1 tbsp lemon juice
• 1 tsp Dijon mustard
• 1 tsp dried dill
• Salt and pepper to taste

Instructions

1. If using wooden skewers, soak them in water for 30 minutes to prevent burning.

2. In a large bowl, combine the shrimp, zucchini pieces, olive oil, lemon juice, oregano, and garlic powder. Season with salt and pepper. Toss to coat everything evenly.

3. Thread the shrimp and zucchini pieces onto the skewers, alternating between the two.

4. Preheat your grill or grill pan to medium•high heat.

5. Grill the shrimp and zucchini skewers for 2•3 minutes per side, or until the shrimp are opaque and the zucchini is tender•crisp.

6. Serve the grilled shrimp and zucchini skewers immediately.

Nutritional Info (per serving):
• Calories: 200
• Total Carbs: 8g
• Fiber: 2g
• Net Carbs: 6g
• Protein: 25g
• Fat: 8g

This grilled shrimp and zucchini skewer dish is an excellent choice for men managing type 2 diabetes. Shrimp is a lean protein that is low in carbs, while zucchini provides fiber and nutrients without significantly impacting blood sugar levels.

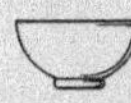 **Preparation Time : 15 min**

 **Total Time : 30 min - 1h**

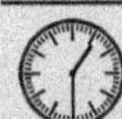 **Servings : 3-6**

Ingredients

• 1 lb large shrimp, peeled and deveined
• 2 medium zucchini, cut into 1•inch pieces
• 2 tbsp olive oil
• 1 tbsp lemon juice
• 1 tsp dried oregano
• 1/2 tsp garlic powder
• Salt and pepper to taste
• Wooden or metal skewers

Instructions

1. In a small bowl, combine the soy sauce, rice vinegar, and sesame oil. Set aside.

2. Heat the olive oil in a large skillet or wok over high heat. Add the chicken and stir•fry for 3•4 minutes until lightly browned.

3. Add the minced garlic and grated ginger to the skillet. Stir•fry for 1 minute until fragrant.

4. Add the broccoli florets and stir•fry for 2•3 minutes.

5. In a small bowl, whisk together the chicken broth and cornstarch. Pour this mixture into the skillet and bring to a simmer.

6. Cook for 2•3 minutes, stirring frequently, until the sauce has thickened and the broccoli is tender•crisp.

7. Remove from heat and stir in the soy sauce mixture. Season with salt and pepper to taste.

8. Serve the chicken and broccoli stir•fry over cooked brown rice, if desired.

Nutritional Info (per serving):
• Calories: 300
• Total Carbs: 12g
• Fiber: 4g
• Net Carbs: 8g
• Protein: 40g
• Fat: 12g

This chicken and broccoli stir•fry is an excellent choice for men managing type 2 diabetes. The lean protein from the chicken, fiber•rich broccoli, and optional brown rice provide a balanced, nutrient•dense meal.

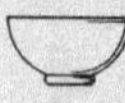 **Preparation Time : 15 min**

 **Total Time : 30 min - 1h**

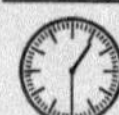 **Servings : 3-6**

Ingredients

• 1 lb boneless, skinless chicken breasts, cut into 1•inch pieces
• 2 tbsp low•sodium soy sauce or tamari
• 1 tbsp rice vinegar
• 1 tsp sesame oil
• 1 tbsp olive oil
• 3 cloves garlic, minced
• 1 inch piece fresh ginger, peeled and grated
• 4 cups broccoli florets
• 1/2 cup low•sodium chicken broth
• 1 tsp cornstarch
• Salt and pepper to taste
• Cooked brown rice, for serving (optional)

Instructions

1. In a large pot or Dutch oven, heat the olive oil over medium heat. Add the diced onion and sauté for 3•4 minutes until translucent.

2. Add the minced garlic, diced bell pepper, and diced jalapeño (if using). Sauté for 2•3 minutes.

3. Stir in the chili powder, cumin, oregano, and cayenne (if using). Cook for 1 minute to toast the spices.

4. Pour in the diced tomatoes, black beans, kidney beans, and vegetable broth. Stir to combine.

5. Bring the chili to a simmer and let it cook for 15•20 minutes, stirring occasionally, until the flavors have melded and the chili has thickened.

6. Season with salt and pepper to taste.

7. Serve the vegetable and bean chili hot, garnished with chopped cilantro if desired.

Nutritional Info (per serving):
• Calories: 250
• Total Carbs: 35g
• Fiber: 12g
• Net Carbs: 23g
• Protein: 12g
• Fat: 6g

This vegetable and bean chili is an excellent choice for men managing type 2 diabetes. The combination of fiber•rich beans, vegetables, and spices provides a nutrient•dense and diabetes•friendly meal.

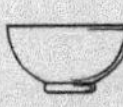 **Preparation Time : 15 min**

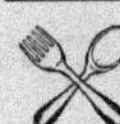 **Total Time : 30 min - 1h**

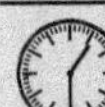 **Servings : 3-6**

Ingredients

• 1 tbsp olive oil
• 1 medium onion, diced
• 3 cloves garlic, minced
• 1 red bell pepper, diced
• 1 jalapeño, seeded and diced (optional)
• 2 tsp chili powder
• 1 tsp ground cumin
• 1 tsp dried oregano
• 1/4 tsp cayenne pepper (optional)
• 1 (15 oz) can diced tomatoes
• 1 (15 oz) can black beans, rinsed and drained
• 1 (15 oz) can kidney beans, rinsed and drained
• 1 cup low•sodium vegetable broth
• Salt and pepper to taste
• Chopped cilantro for garnish (optional)

Instructions

1. Preheat oven to 400°F. Line a large baking sheet with parchment paper.

2. Place the cod fillets on one side of the prepared baking sheet. Arrange the trimmed and halved Brussels sprouts on the other side of the sheet.

3. In a small bowl, whisk together the olive oil, lemon juice, Dijon mustard, and dried thyme. Season with a pinch of salt and pepper.

4. Drizzle the oil and lemon mixture evenly over the cod and Brussels sprouts, making sure to coat everything.

5. Bake for 15•18 minutes, or until the cod is cooked through and flakes easily with a fork, and the Brussels sprouts are tender and lightly browned.

6. Serve the baked cod and Brussels sprouts immediately.

Nutritional Info (per serving):
• Calories: 280
• Total Carbs: 12g
• Fiber: 5g
• Net Carbs: 7g
• Protein: 35g
• Fat: 12g

This baked cod and Brussels sprouts dish is an excellent choice for men managing type 2 diabetes. Cod is a lean, high•protein fish, while Brussels sprouts provide fiber, vitamins, and minerals.

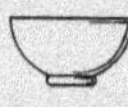 **Preparation Time : 15 min**

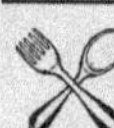 **Total Time : 30 min - 1h**

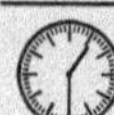 **Servings : 3-6**

Ingredients

• 4 (6 oz) cod fillets
• 1 lb Brussels sprouts, trimmed and halved
• 2 tbsp olive oil
• 1 tbsp lemon juice
• 1 tsp Dijon mustard
• 1 tsp dried thyme
• Salt and pepper to taste

Instructions

1. Preheat oven to 400°F. Line a baking sheet with parchment paper.

2. In a medium bowl, combine the ground turkey, breadcrumbs, egg, Parmesan, garlic, oregano, and red pepper flakes (if using). Season with salt and pepper. Mix well until fully incorporated.

3. Roll the turkey mixture into 1•inch meatballs and place them on the prepared baking sheet.

4. Bake the meatballs for 18•20 minutes, until cooked through.

5. While the meatballs are baking, prepare the zucchini noodles.

6. In a large skillet, heat the marinara sauce over medium heat. Add the zucchini noodles and toss to coat, cooking for 2•3 minutes until the noodles are tender but still crisp.

7. Serve the zucchini noodles topped with the baked turkey meatballs.

Nutritional Info (per serving):
• Calories: 300
• Total Carbs: 15g
• Fiber: 4g
• Net Carbs: 11g
• Protein: 30g
• Fat: 12g

This turkey meatball and zucchini noodle dish is an excellent choice for men managing type 2 diabetes. The lean turkey provides protein, while the zucchini noodles offer a low•carb, fiber•rich alternative to traditional pasta.

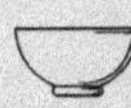 **Preparation Time : 15 min**

 **Total Time : 30 min - 1h**

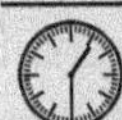 **Servings : 3-6**

Ingredients

• 1 lb ground turkey
• 1/4 cup whole wheat breadcrumbs
• 1 egg, lightly beaten
• 2 tbsp grated Parmesan cheese
• 2 cloves garlic, minced
• 1 tsp dried oregano
• 1/4 tsp red pepper flakes (optional)
• Salt and pepper to taste
• 3 medium zucchini, spiralized or julienned into noodles
• 1 cup marinara sauce (no•sugar•added)

27. Grilled Portobello Mushrooms with Quinoa

Instructions

1. Preheat grill or grill pan to medium·high heat.

2. In a shallow dish, combine the olive oil, balsamic vinegar, thyme, salt, and pepper. Add the mushroom caps and turn to coat both sides.

3. Grill the mushrooms for 4·5 minutes per side, until tender and slightly charred.

4. Remove the mushrooms from the grill and place on a serving plate.

5. In a small bowl, mix together the cooked quinoa, feta cheese, and chopped parsley.

6. Spoon the quinoa mixture into the center of each grilled mushroom cap.

7. Serve the stuffed mushrooms immediately, while warm.

Enjoy this healthy and flavorful grilled portobello dish! The meaty mushrooms pair perfectly with the nutty quinoa and tangy feta.

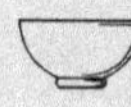 **Preparation Time : 15 min**

 **Total Time : 30 min - 1h**

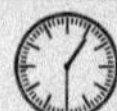 **Servings : 3-6**

Ingredients

- 4 large portobello mushroom caps, stems removed
- 2 tbsp olive oil
- 1 tsp balsamic vinegar
- 1 tsp dried thyme
- Salt and pepper to taste
- 1 cup cooked quinoa
- 2 tbsp crumbled feta cheese
- 2 tbsp chopped fresh parsley

Instructions

1. Preheat oven to 400°F. Lightly grease a baking dish or line a baking sheet with parchment paper.

2. Using a sharp knife, carefully slice a pocket into the side of each chicken breast, being careful not to cut all the way through.

3. In a small bowl, mix together the chopped spinach and crumbled feta cheese.

4. Stuff the spinach and feta mixture evenly into the pockets of the chicken breasts.

5. Drizzle the olive oil over the top of the stuffed chicken breasts and sprinkle with the dried oregano. Season with salt and pepper.

6. Bake for 25•30 minutes, or until the chicken is cooked through and the internal temperature reaches 165°F.

7. Let the stuffed chicken breasts rest for 5 minutes before serving.

Nutritional Info (per serving):
• Calories: 280
• Total Carbs: 3g
• Fiber: 1g
• Net Carbs: 2g
• Protein: 40g
• Fat: 12g

This stuffed chicken breast dish is an excellent choice for men managing type 2 diabetes. The lean chicken breast provides a good source of protein, while the spinach and feta cheese add flavor and nutrients without significantly impacting carbohydrate intake.

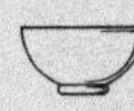 **Preparation Time : 15 min**

 **Total Time : 30 min - 1h**

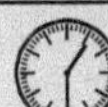 **Servings : 3-6**

Ingredients

• 4 (6 oz) boneless, skinless chicken breasts
• 1 cup fresh spinach, chopped
• 1/4 cup crumbled feta cheese
• 1 tbsp olive oil
• 1 tsp dried oregano
• Salt and pepper to taste

Instructions

1. If using wooden skewers, soak them in water for 30 minutes to prevent burning.

2. In a large bowl, combine the beef cubes, bell pepper, zucchini, onion, and mushrooms.

3. In a small bowl, whisk together the olive oil, balsamic vinegar, oregano, and garlic powder. Season with salt and pepper.

4. Pour the marinade over the beef and vegetables and toss to coat everything evenly.

5. Thread the marinated beef and vegetables onto the skewers, alternating the ingredients.

6. Preheat your grill or grill pan to medium•high heat.

7. Grill the kebabs for 10•12 minutes, turning occasionally, until the beef is cooked through and the vegetables are tender•crisp.

8. Serve the grilled beef and vegetable kebabs immediately.

Nutritional Info (per serving):
• Calories: 250
• Total Carbs: 10g
• Fiber: 3g
• Net Carbs: 7g
• Protein: 25g
• Fat: 12g

These beef and vegetable kebabs are an excellent choice for men managing type 2 diabetes. The lean beef provides protein, while the variety of vegetables add fiber, vitamins, and minerals.

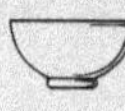 **Preparation Time : 15 min**

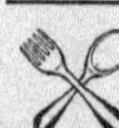 **Total Time : 30 min - 1h**

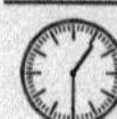 **Servings : 3-6**

Ingredients

• 1 lb beef sirloin or tenderloin, cut into 1•inch cubes
• 1 red bell pepper, cut into 1•inch pieces
• 1 zucchini, cut into 1•inch pieces
• 1 red onion, cut into 1•inch pieces
• 8 oz mushrooms, halved
• 2 tbsp olive oil
• 1 tbsp balsamic vinegar
• 1 tsp dried oregano
• 1/2 tsp garlic powder
• Salt and pepper to taste
• Wooden or metal skewers

Instructions

1. Preheat oven to 375°F. Line a baking sheet with parchment paper.

2. In a shallow bowl, combine the whole wheat breadcrumbs, Parmesan cheese, oregano, garlic powder, and red pepper flakes (if using).

3. Dip the eggplant slices into the beaten eggs, then coat them in the breadcrumb mixture, pressing gently to adhere.

4. Arrange the breaded eggplant slices in a single layer on the prepared baking sheet.

5. Bake for 20•25 minutes, flipping the slices halfway, until the eggplant is tender and the breadcrumbs are golden brown.

6. Spread 1/2 cup of the marinara sauce in the bottom of a baking dish. Arrange the baked eggplant slices in a single layer over the sauce.

7. Top the eggplant with the remaining 1/2 cup of marinara sauce and the shredded mozzarella cheese.

8. Bake for an additional 15•20 minutes, until the cheese is melted and bubbly.

9. Let the eggplant parmesan cool for 5 minutes before serving.

This eggplant parmesan dish is a great option for men managing type 2 diabetes. The whole wheat breadcrumbs provide complex carbs and fiber, while the eggplant, marinara sauce, and mozzarella cheese create a satisfying and diabetes•friendly meal.

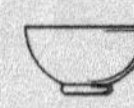 **Preparation Time : 15 min**

 **Total Time : 30 min - 1h**

 **Servings : 3-6**

Ingredients

• 1 medium eggplant, sliced into 1/2•inch rounds
• 1 cup whole wheat breadcrumbs
• 1/2 cup grated Parmesan cheese
• 1 tsp dried oregano
• 1/2 tsp garlic powder
• 1/4 tsp red pepper flakes (optional)
• 2 eggs, beaten
• 1 cup marinara sauce (no•sugar•added)
• 1 cup shredded part•skim mozzarella cheese

Instructions

1. Wash and core the apples. Slice them into thin wedges or slices.

2. Arrange the apple slices on a plate or platter.

3. Serve the almond butter in a small bowl or ramekin alongside the apple slices.

4. Encourage the person to dip the apple slices into the almond butter as a healthy snack.

This snack is an excellent choice for men managing type 2 diabetes for a few reasons:

1. Apples are a low•glycemic fruit, meaning they won't cause a rapid spike in blood sugar levels. They are high in fiber, which helps regulate blood sugar.

2. Almond butter is a great source of healthy monounsaturated fats, protein, and fiber. The combination of the apple and almond butter provides a balanced snack that can help keep blood sugar stable.

3. The fiber, protein, and healthy fats in this snack help promote feelings of fullness and satisfaction, which can prevent overeating.

4. This snack is easy to prepare and portable, making it a convenient option for managing diabetes on•the•go.

Encourage the person to enjoy this snack as part of a balanced, diabetes•friendly diet. The combination of the apple and almond butter provides a nutritious and delicious way to satisfy hunger while keeping blood sugar in check.

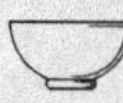 **Preparation Time : 15 min**

 **Total Time : 30 min - 1h**

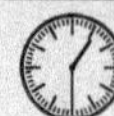 **Servings : 3-6**

Ingredients

• 2 medium apples, cored and sliced
• 1/4 cup natural almond butter (no added sugar)

Instructions

1. Make the hummus (if making homemade):
   • In a food processor, combine the chickpeas, tahini, lemon juice, garlic, olive oil, cumin, and paprika. Blend until smooth.
   • Season with salt and pepper to taste.

2. Prepare the carrot and celery sticks:
   • Wash and peel the carrots. Cut them into long, thin sticks.
   • Wash the celery stalks and cut them into 4•inch sticks.

3. Arrange the carrot and celery sticks on a serving platter.

4. Serve the hummus alongside the vegetable sticks.

This snack is an excellent choice for men managing type 2 diabetes. The carrot and celery sticks provide fiber, vitamins, and minerals, while the hummus offers protein, healthy fats, and complex carbohydrates. The combination helps to regulate blood sugar levels and provide a satisfying, nutrient•dense snack.

Enjoy this simple and delicious diabetic•friendly snack!

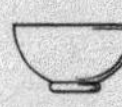 **Preparation Time : 15 min**

 **Total Time : 30 min - 1h**

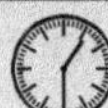 **Servings : 3-6**

Ingredients

• 4 medium carrots, peeled and cut into sticks
• 4 celery stalks, cut into sticks
• 1 cup homemade or store•bought hummus

For the Hummus:
• 1 (15 oz) can chickpeas, drained and rinsed
• 2 tbsp tahini
• 2 tbsp fresh lemon juice
• 1 garlic clove, minced
• 2 tbsp olive oil
• 1/4 tsp ground cumin
• 1/4 tsp paprika
• Salt and pepper to taste

Instructions

1. In a medium bowl, combine the Greek yogurt, diced cucumber, chopped dill, garlic powder, salt, and black pepper. Stir until well mixed.

2. Serve the yogurt mixture immediately or refrigerate until ready to serve.

This snack is an excellent choice for men managing type 2 diabetes for several reasons:

1. Greek yogurt is high in protein and low in carbohydrates, which helps regulate blood sugar levels.

2. Cucumbers are a low•calorie, low•carb vegetable that provides hydration and fiber.

3. Dill is a flavorful herb that can help reduce inflammation and may have a positive impact on blood sugar control.

4. The combination of the protein•rich yogurt, fiber•filled cucumber, and anti•inflammatory dill creates a balanced, diabetes•friendly snack.

Encourage the person to enjoy this snack as part of a healthy, balanced diet. The Greek yogurt, cucumber, and dill provide a refreshing and nutritious option that can help manage type 2 diabetes.

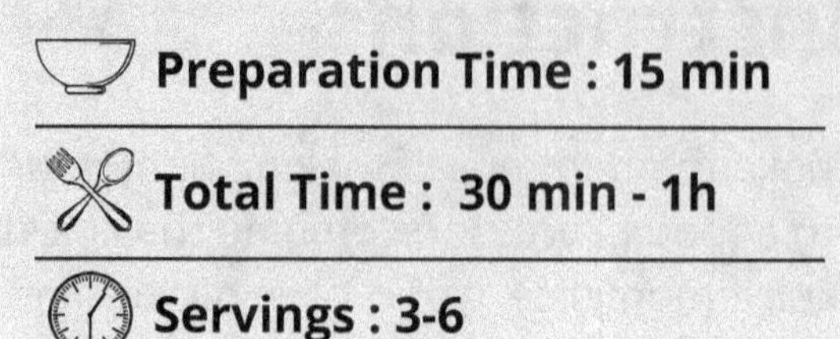

Preparation Time : 15 min

Total Time : 30 min - 1h

Servings : 3-6

Ingredients

• 1 cup plain, unsweetened Greek yogurt
• 1/2 cup diced cucumber
• 1 tbsp chopped fresh dill
• 1/4 tsp garlic powder
• 1/4 tsp salt
• 1/8 tsp black pepper

Instructions

1. Preheat oven to 325°F (165°C).

2. In a large bowl, combine the almonds, cashews, walnuts, pumpkin seeds, and sunflower seeds.

3. Drizzle the olive oil over the nut and seed mixture and toss to coat evenly.

4. In a small bowl, mix together the cumin, smoked paprika, garlic powder, and cayenne pepper (if using).

5. Sprinkle the spice mixture over the nut and seed mixture and toss to coat evenly.

6. Spread the seasoned nuts and seeds in a single layer on a large baking sheet.

7. Bake for 12•15 minutes, stirring halfway, until lightly toasted and fragrant.

8. Remove from oven and sprinkle with sea salt. Toss to coat.

9. Allow the mixed nuts and seeds to cool completely before serving.

Store in an airtight container at room temperature for up to 2 weeks.

Enjoy this flavorful and nutritious snack mix! The combination of nuts and seeds provides a great source of healthy fats, protein, and fiber.

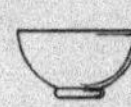 **Preparation Time : 15 min**

 **Total Time : 30 min - 1h**

 **Servings : 3-6**

Ingredients

- 1 cup raw almonds
- 1 cup raw cashews
- 1 cup raw walnuts
- 1/2 cup raw pumpkin seeds
- 1/2 cup raw sunflower seeds
- 1 tbsp olive oil
- 1 tsp ground cumin
- 1 tsp smoked paprika
- 1 tsp garlic powder
- 1/2 tsp cayenne pepper (optional for spicy)
- 1 tsp sea salt

Instructions

1. Make the guacamole:
   • In a medium bowl, gently mash the diced avocados with a fork.
   • Stir in the lime juice, red onion, garlic, cilantro, salt, and cumin. Mix well until combined.
   • Taste and adjust seasoning as needed.

2. Prepare the bell pepper strips:
   • Wash the bell peppers and slice them into long, thin strips.

3. Serve the guacamole in a small bowl, surrounded by the bell pepper strips.

This snack is a great option for anyone looking for a healthy, flavorful, and nutrient•dense option. The bell pepper strips provide a crunchy vehicle for the creamy, savory guacamole.

Some key benefits of this snack:

• Bell peppers are low in calories and carbohydrates, making them a great choice for those managing their blood sugar levels.
• Avocados are rich in healthy monounsaturated fats, fiber, and various vitamins and minerals.
• The combination of the bell peppers and guacamole provides a good source of antioxidants, vitamins, and fiber.
• This snack is easy to prepare and can be enjoyed as a quick, satisfying, and nutritious option.

Encourage the person to enjoy this snack as part of a balanced, diabetes•friendly diet. The bell pepper strips and guacamole make for a delicious and healthy pairing.

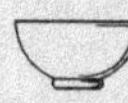 **Preparation Time : 15 min**

 **Total Time : 30 min - 1h**

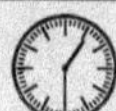 **Servings : 3-6**

Ingredients

For the Guacamole:
• 2 ripe avocados, pitted and diced
• 1 tablespoon fresh lime juice
• 2 tablespoons diced red onion
• 1 garlic clove, minced
• 2 tablespoons chopped cilantro
• 1/4 teaspoon salt
• 1/8 teaspoon ground cumin

For the Bell Pepper Strips:
• 2 large bell peppers (any color), washed and cut into long, thin strips

Instructions

1. Place the eggs in a single layer in a saucepan and cover with cold water by 1 inch.

2. Bring the water to a boil over high heat.

3. Once the water reaches a rolling boil, remove the pan from the heat and cover with a lid.

4. Let the eggs sit in the hot water for 12 minutes for hard•boiled eggs.

5. Drain the hot water and cover the eggs with cold water to stop the cooking process.

6. Let the eggs sit in the cold water for 5 minutes.

7. Peel the eggs and enjoy as a snack or use in other recipes.

Hard•boiled eggs are an excellent snack choice for men managing type 2 diabetes for the following reasons:

1. Eggs are a high•quality source of protein, which can help regulate blood sugar levels and promote feelings of fullness.

2. The protein in eggs does not contain any carbohydrates, making them a low•glycemic food that won't spike blood sugar.

3. Hard•boiled eggs are a convenient, portable, and easy•to•prepare snack that can be kept on hand for quick access.

4. Eggs are a versatile ingredient that can be incorporated into a variety of diabetes•friendly meals and snacks.

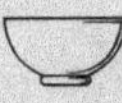 **Preparation Time : 15 min**

 **Total Time : 30 min - 1h**

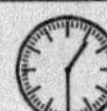 **Servings : 3-6**

Ingredients

• 6 large eggs

5. The preparation method of hard•boiling the eggs does not require any added fats, oils, or seasonings that could potentially impact blood sugar control.

Encourage the person to enjoy hard•boiled eggs as a nutritious snack option, and provide guidance on appropriate portion sizes and the importance of incorporating a variety of protein sources into their diet to manage type 2 diabetes effectively.

Instructions

1. Bring a large pot of water to a boil.

2. Add the frozen edamame pods to the boiling water and cook for 5•7 minutes, or until the pods are bright green and tender.

3. Drain the edamame and transfer to a serving bowl.

4. Sprinkle the sea salt over the edamame and toss to coat.

5. Serve the edamame warm, providing a small bowl for the empty pods.

Edamame is an excellent snack choice for men managing type 2 diabetes for the following reasons:

1. Edamame is a low•glycemic food, meaning it won't cause a rapid spike in blood sugar levels. The fiber and protein in edamame help slow the absorption of carbohydrates.

2. Edamame is a good source of plant•based protein, which can help promote feelings of fullness and satisfaction, preventing overeating.

3. The fiber in edamame can help improve digestion and regulate bowel movements, which is important for overall health in those with diabetes.

4. Edamame is low in calories and contains no added sugars or unhealthy fats, making it a diabetes•friendly snack option.

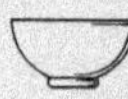 **Preparation Time : 15 min**

 **Total Time : 30 min - 1h**

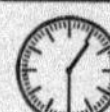 **Servings : 3-6**

Ingredients

- 1 lb frozen edamame in the pod
- 1 tsp sea salt (or to taste)

5. The simple preparation of boiling and seasoning with salt allows the natural flavors of the edamame to shine, without the need for any additional sauces or seasonings that may contain added sugars.

Encourage the person to enjoy edamame as a healthy, portable, and satisfying snack that can help manage their type 2 diabetes. Provide guidance on appropriate portion sizes and the importance of incorporating a variety of nutrient•dense foods into their diet.

Instructions

1. Select whole grain crackers that are high in fiber and low in added sugars and refined carbohydrates. Some good options include:
   • Whole wheat crackers
   • Multigrain crackers
   • Rye crackers
   • Seed crackers

2. Choose a low•fat or reduced•fat cheese variety. Good options include:
   • Cheddar cheese
   • Swiss cheese
   • Cottage cheese
   • Mozzarella cheese

3. Arrange the whole grain crackers on a plate or platter.

4. Top each cracker with a small slice or portion of the selected cheese.

Encourage the person to pay attention to portion sizes and to choose whole grain crackers and low•fat cheese varieties to keep this snack diabetes•friendly. Enjoy this snack as part of a balanced, healthy diet.

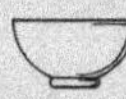 **Preparation Time : 15 min**

 **Total Time : 30 min - 1h**

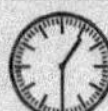 **Servings : 3-6**

Ingredients

• 8•10 whole grain crackers (look for ones with at least 3g of fiber per serving)
• 1•2 oz of low•fat or reduced•fat cheese (such as cheddar, Swiss, or cottage cheese)

This snack is an excellent choice for men managing type 2 diabetes for several reasons:

1. Whole grain crackers are a complex carbohydrate that is digested more slowly, helping to prevent blood sugar spikes.
2. The fiber in the whole grain crackers helps promote feelings of fullness and can improve digestion.
3. Low•fat or reduced•fat cheese provides protein, which can also help regulate blood sugar levels and keep you feeling satisfied.
4. The combination of the complex carbs from the crackers and the protein from the cheese creates a balanced snack.
5. This snack is easy to prepare and portable, making it a convenient option for managing diabetes on•the•go.

Instructions

1. Rinse and gently pat dry the mixed berries.
2. Place the berries in a serving bowl or dish.
3. Sprinkle the chia seeds evenly over the top of the berries.

This snack is an excellent choice for men managing type 2 diabetes for several reasons:

1. Berries are a low•glycemic fruit, meaning they won't cause a rapid spike in blood sugar levels. They are high in fiber, vitamins, and antioxidants.

2. Chia seeds are a great source of fiber, protein, and healthy omega•3 fatty acids. The fiber and protein in chia seeds can help slow the absorption of carbohydrates, preventing blood sugar spikes.

3. The combination of the low•glycemic berries and the fiber•rich chia seeds creates a balanced, diabetes•friendly snack that can help regulate blood sugar levels.

4. This snack is easy to prepare, portable, and requires no cooking, making it a convenient option for managing diabetes on•the•go.

5. Berries and chia seeds are low in calories and contain no added sugars or unhealthy fats, making them a nutritious choice for those with type 2 diabetes.

Encourage the person to enjoy this snack as part of a balanced, diabetes•friendly diet. Provide guidance on appropriate portion sizes and the importance of incorporating a variety of nutrient•dense foods into their daily routine to effectively manage type 2 diabetes.

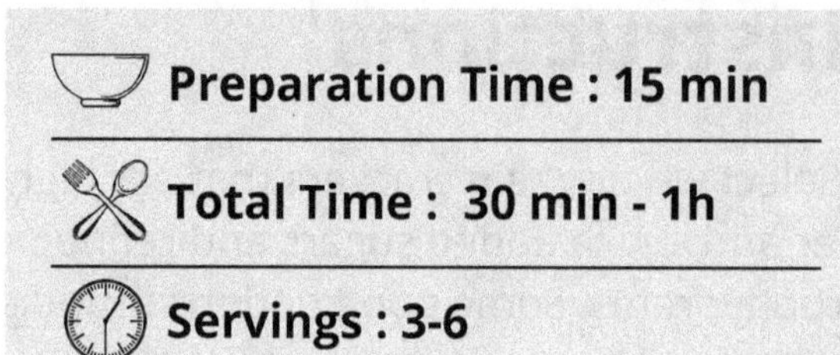

Ingredients

• 1 cup mixed berries (such as blueberries, raspberries, blackberries)
• 1 tbsp chia seeds

Instructions

1. Preheat your oven to 400°F (200°C).

2. Drain and rinse the chickpeas, then pat them dry with a paper towel or clean kitchen towel.

3. In a medium bowl, toss the chickpeas with the olive oil, cumin, paprika, garlic powder, salt, and black pepper until they are evenly coated.

4. Spread the seasoned chickpeas in a single layer on a baking sheet lined with parchment paper.

5. Roast the chickpeas in the preheated oven for 20•25 minutes, stirring halfway, until they are crispy and golden brown.

6. Remove the roasted chickpeas from the oven and let them cool for a few minutes before serving.

Roasted chickpeas make an excellent snack for men managing type 2 diabetes for several reasons:

1. Chickpeas are a good source of fiber, protein, and complex carbohydrates, which can help regulate blood sugar levels.
2. The roasting process helps reduce the glycemic index of the chickpeas, further slowing the release of sugars into the bloodstream.
3. The spices used (cumin, paprika, and garlic) add flavor without the need for added sugars or salt, which can be problematic for those with diabetes.
4. Roasted chickpeas are a crunchy, satisfying snack that can help curb hunger and prevent overeating.

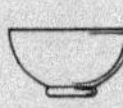 **Preparation Time : 15 min**

 **Total Time : 30 min - 1h**

 **Servings : 3-6**

Ingredients

- 1 (15 oz) can chickpeas (garbanzo beans), drained and rinsed
- 1 tbsp olive oil
- 1 tsp ground cumin
- 1 tsp paprika
- 1/2 tsp garlic powder
- 1/4 tsp salt
- 1/4 tsp black pepper

Encourage the person to enjoy these roasted chickpeas as a healthy, diabetes•friendly snack option. They can be stored in an airtight container for up to 1 week, making them a convenient and nutritious choice.

Instructions

1. Line a baking sheet or plate with parchment paper.

2. In a small, microwave•safe bowl, melt the chopped dark chocolate in the microwave, stirring every 30 seconds, until smooth and fully melted.

3. Holding them by the stem, dip each strawberry into the melted dark chocolate, coating about 3/4 of the berry.

4. Gently tap off any excess chocolate and place the dipped strawberries on the prepared baking sheet or plate.

5. Refrigerate the chocolate•covered strawberries for at least 30 minutes, or until the chocolate has hardened. Serve chilled.

This dark chocolate•covered strawberry treat is an excellent option for men managing type 2 diabetes for several reasons:

1. Strawberries are a low•glycemic fruit, meaning they won't cause a rapid spike in blood sugar levels.
2. Dark chocolate with a high cacao content is lower in sugar and higher in antioxidants compared to milk chocolate.
3. The combination of the fruit and dark chocolate provides a satisfying, sweet treat without overwhelming the body with carbohydrates.
4. The portion size of 1•2 strawberries per serving helps to control calorie and carbohydrate intake.
5. This snack is easy to prepare and can be enjoyed as an occasional indulgence as part of a balanced, diabetes•friendly diet

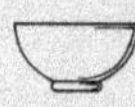 **Preparation Time : 15 min**

 **Total Time : 30 min - 1h**

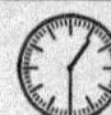 **Servings : 3-6**

Ingredients

• 12 fresh strawberries, washed and patted dry
• 2 oz dark chocolate (at least 70% cacao), chopped

Encourage the person to choose dark chocolate with a cacao content of at least 70% and to limit their portion size to 1•2 strawberries. Remind them that even healthy treats should be consumed in moderation when managing type 2 diabetes.

42. Greek Yogurt with Honey and Almonds

Instructions

1. Scoop the Greek yogurt into a serving bowl.

2. Drizzle the honey over the top of the yogurt.

3. Sprinkle the sliced or slivered almonds over the honey•topped yogurt.

4. Serve immediately.

This snack is an excellent choice for men managing type 2 diabetes for the following reasons:

1. Greek yogurt is high in protein and low in carbohydrates, which helps regulate blood sugar levels.

2. Honey is a natural sweetener that has a lower glycemic index compared to refined sugar, making it a better option for those with diabetes.

3. Almonds are a source of healthy fats, fiber, and protein, which can help slow the absorption of carbohydrates and promote feelings of fullness.

4. The combination of the protein•rich yogurt, natural sweetener, and nutrient•dense almonds creates a balanced, diabetes•friendly snack.

5. This snack is easy to prepare, portable, and can be enjoyed as a quick, satisfying option.

Encourage the person to use a small portion of honey, as even natural sweeteners should be consumed in moderation when managing type 2 diabetes. Provide guidance on appropriate serving sizes and the importance of incorporating a variety of nutrient•dense foods into their diet.

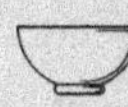 **Preparation Time : 15 min**

 **Total Time : 30 min - 1h**

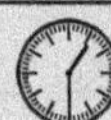 **Servings : 3-6**

Ingredients

- 1 cup plain, unsweetened Greek yogurt
- 1 tbsp raw, unprocessed honey
- 2 tbsp sliced or slivered almonds

Instructions

1. In a medium bowl, whisk together the chia seeds, almond milk, honey (or sweetener), and vanilla extract until well combined.

2. Cover the bowl and refrigerate for at least 2 hours, or overnight, stirring occasionally, until the chia seeds have thickened the mixture into a pudding•like consistency.

3. When ready to serve, stir the chia seed pudding to ensure it is smooth and creamy.

4. Divide the chia seed pudding into individual serving bowls or cups.

5. Top each serving with 1/4 cup of diced fresh mango.

6. Serve chilled.

This chia seed pudding with mango is an excellent snack choice for men managing type 2 diabetes for the following reasons:

1. Chia seeds are high in fiber, protein, and healthy omega•3 fatty acids, which can help regulate blood sugar levels.
2. Unsweetened almond milk is low in carbohydrates and provides a creamy base for the pudding.
3. Honey is used as a natural sweetener, which has a lower glycemic index compared to refined sugar.
4. Mango is a low•glycemic fruit that provides vitamins, minerals, and fiber.
5. The combination of the nutrient•dense chia seeds, low•carb milk, and fresh fruit creates a balanced, diabetes•friendly snack.

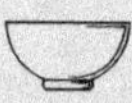 **Preparation Time : 15 min**

 **Total Time : 30 min - 1h**

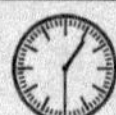 **Servings : 3-6**

Ingredients

• 1/4 cup chia seeds
• 1 cup unsweetened almond milk (or other non•dairy milk)
• 1 tbsp honey (or 1•2 tsp zero•calorie sweetener)
• 1/2 tsp vanilla extract
• 1 cup diced fresh mango

Encourage the person to use a small amount of honey or a zero•calorie sweetener to control the overall carbohydrate content. Portion control is also important, as even healthy snacks should be consumed in moderation as part of a balanced, diabetes•friendly diet.

Instructions

1. Preheat your oven to 375°F (190°C).

2. Core the apples and cut them in half horizontally. Place the apple halves in a baking dish or on a parchment•lined baking sheet.

3. Sprinkle the ground cinnamon evenly over the top of the apple halves.

4. (Optional) Spoon a small amount of unsweetened applesauce into the center of each apple half.

5. Bake the apples for 20•25 minutes, or until they are tender and easily pierced with a fork.

6. Remove the baked apples from the oven and let them cool for a few minutes before serving.

This baked apple dish is an excellent snack choice for men managing type 2 diabetes for the following reasons:

1. Apples are a low•glycemic fruit, meaning they won't cause a rapid spike in blood sugar levels. They are high in fiber, which helps regulate blood sugar.

2. Cinnamon has been shown to have a positive effect on blood sugar control and insulin sensitivity.

3. The baking process helps to concentrate the natural sweetness of the apples, reducing the need for added sugars.

4. The optional applesauce provides a touch of extra moisture and flavor without significantly increasing the carbohydrate content.

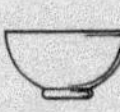 **Preparation Time : 15 min**

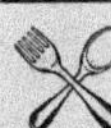 **Total Time : 30 min - 1h**

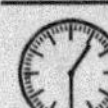 **Servings : 3-6**

Ingredients

• 2 medium•sized apples, cored and halved
• 2 tsp ground cinnamon
• 1 tbsp unsweetened applesauce (optional)

5. This snack is easy to prepare, satisfying, and provides a sweet, comforting treat without compromising blood sugar management.

Encourage the person to enjoy this baked apple snack as part of a balanced, diabetes•friendly diet. Provide guidance on appropriate portion sizes and the importance of incorporating a variety of fruits and vegetables into their daily routine.

45. Mixed Berries with a Dollop of Whipped Cream

Instructions

1. Rinse and gently pat dry the mixed berries.
2. Place the berries in a serving bowl or dish.
3. Top the berries with a small dollop (about 2 tbsp) of unsweetened whipped cream.

This snack is an excellent choice for men managing type 2 diabetes for the following reasons:

1. Berries are a low•glycemic fruit, meaning they won't cause a rapid spike in blood sugar levels. They are high in fiber, vitamins, and antioxidants.

2. Unsweetened whipped cream is low in carbohydrates and provides a creamy, satisfying complement to the berries.

3. The combination of the low•glycemic berries and the healthy fats from the whipped cream creates a balanced snack that can help regulate blood sugar levels.

4. This snack is easy to prepare, portable, and requires no cooking, making it a convenient option for managing diabetes on•the•go.

5. The portion size of 1 cup of berries with a small dollop of whipped cream is a reasonable, diabetes•friendly serving.

Encourage the person to use unsweetened whipped cream and to be mindful of portion sizes, as even healthy fats should be consumed in moderation when managing type 2 diabetes. This snack can be enjoyed as part of a balanced, diabetes•friendly diet.

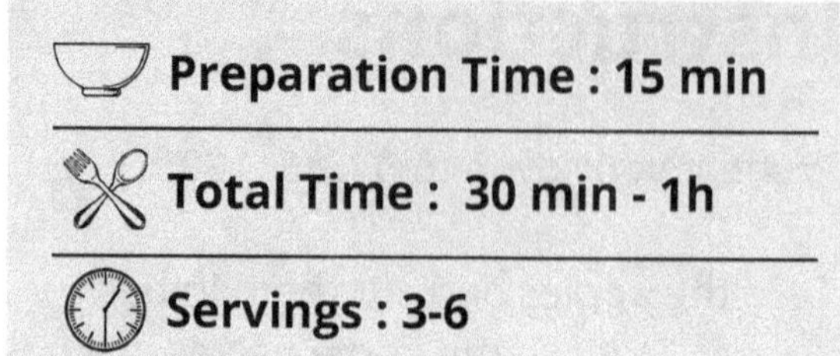

Preparation Time : 15 min

Total Time : 30 min - 1h

Servings : 3-6

Ingredients

• 1 cup mixed berries (such as blueberries, raspberries, and blackberries)
• 2 tbsp unsweetened whipped cream

Instructions

1. Preheat your oven to 350°F (175°C). Grease an 8x8•inch baking pan with coconut oil or non•stick cooking spray.

2. In a medium bowl, whisk together the coconut flour, cocoa powder, baking soda, and salt.

3. In a separate bowl, beat the eggs and erythritol (or other sweetener) until well combined.

4. Stir in the melted coconut oil (or butter) and vanilla extract.

5. Gradually add the dry ingredients to the wet ingredients, mixing until just combined. Do not overmix.

6. Spread the batter evenly into the prepared baking pan.

7. Bake for 18•22 minutes, or until a toothpick inserted in the center comes out clean.

8. Allow the brownies to cool completely before cutting into squares.

Encourage the person to enjoy these brownies in moderation as part of a balanced, diabetes•friendly diet. Portion control is key, as even low•carb treats should be consumed mindfully.

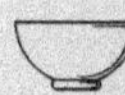 **Preparation Time : 15 min**

 **Total Time : 30 min - 1h**

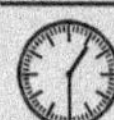 **Servings : 3-6**

Ingredients

- 1/2 cup coconut flour
- 1/4 cup unsweetened cocoa powder
- 1/4 tsp baking soda
- 1/4 tsp salt
- 3 large eggs
- 1/3 cup granulated erythritol or other zero•calorie sweetener
- 1/4 cup melted coconut oil or unsalted butter
- 1 tsp vanilla extract

These coconut flour brownies are an excellent treat option for men managing type 2 diabetes for several reasons:

1. Coconut flour is low in carbohydrates and high in fiber, which helps regulate blood sugar levels.
2. Erythritol is a zero•calorie sweetener that does not impact blood sugar.
3. The high•fat content from the coconut oil or butter helps provide a satisfying, filling dessert.
4. The small portion size and low•carb ingredients make these brownies a diabetes•friendly indulgence.

Instructions

1. Line a baking sheet or plate with parchment paper.

2. Spread the peanut butter evenly on one side of each banana slice.

3. Place the peanut butter•topped banana slices on the prepared baking sheet or plate.

4. Sprinkle the unsweetened shredded coconut over the peanut butter, if using.

5. Freeze the banana bites for at least 2 hours, or until completely frozen.

6. Once frozen, transfer the banana bites to an airtight container or resealable bag and store in the freezer until ready to serve.

This frozen banana bite snack is an excellent choice for men managing type 2 diabetes for the following reasons:

1. Bananas are a source of fiber, potassium, and complex carbohydrates, which can help regulate blood sugar levels.
2. Natural peanut butter provides healthy fats and protein to help slow the absorption of carbohydrates.
3. The freezing process helps to reduce the glycemic impact of the banana, while still providing a sweet and satisfying treat.
4. The optional unsweetened coconut adds a touch of healthy fat and fiber without significantly increasing the carbohydrate content.
5. This snack is easy to prepare, portable, and can be enjoyed as an occasional indulgence as part of a balanced, diabetes•friendly diet.

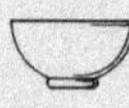 **Preparation Time : 15 min**

 **Total Time : 30 min - 1h**

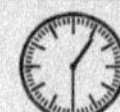 **Servings : 3-6**

Ingredients

• 2 ripe bananas, peeled and cut into 1•inch slices
• 2 tbsp natural peanut butter (no added sugar)
• 1 tbsp unsweetened shredded coconut (optional)

Encourage the person to use natural peanut butter without added sugars and to be mindful of portion sizes, as even healthy fats should be consumed in moderation when managing type 2 diabetes. This frozen banana bite snack can be a delicious and diabetes•friendly option.

Instructions

1. Preheat your oven to 350°F (175°C). Line a baking sheet with parchment paper.

2. In a medium bowl, whisk together the almond flour, erythritol (or other sweetener), salt, and baking soda.

3. In a separate bowl, beat the softened butter until creamy. Add the egg and vanilla extract, and mix until well combined.

4. Gradually add the dry ingredients to the wet ingredients, mixing until a dough forms.

5. Scoop the dough by the tablespoonful and place the balls of dough onto the prepared baking sheet, spacing them about 2 inches apart.

6. Gently flatten each cookie with the back of a fork.

7. Bake for 10•12 minutes, or until the cookies are lightly golden around the edges.

8. Remove the cookies from the oven and let them cool on the baking sheet for 5 minutes before transferring to a wire rack to cool completely.

Encourage the person to enjoy these cookies in moderation as part of a balanced, diabetes•friendly diet. Portion control is key, as even low•carb treats should be consumed mindfully.

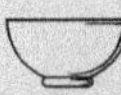 **Preparation Time : 15 min**

 **Total Time : 30 min - 1h**

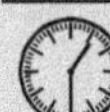 **Servings : 3-6**

Ingredients

• 2 cups almond flour
• 1/4 cup granulated erythritol or other zero•calorie sweetener
• 1/4 tsp salt
• 1/4 tsp baking soda
• 1/4 cup unsalted butter, softened
• 1 large egg
• 1 tsp vanilla extract

These almond flour cookies are an excellent treat option for men managing type 2 diabetes for several reasons:

1. Almond flour is low in carbohydrates and high in healthy fats and fiber, which can help regulate blood sugar levels.
2. Erythritol is a zero•calorie sweetener that does not impact blood sugar.
3. The small portion size and low•carb ingredients make these cookies a diabetes•friendly indulgence.
4. The cookies are easy to prepare and can satisfy a sweet craving without compromising blood sugar control.

Instructions

1. In a medium saucepan, bring the 1 cup of water to a boil.

2. Remove the saucepan from the heat and stir in the package of sugar•free Jello powder until it is completely dissolved.

3. Pour the Jello mixture into a serving bowl or individual ramekins.

4. Refrigerate the Jello for at least 4 hours, or until it is fully set.

5. Once the Jello is set, top it with the fresh or frozen fruit. Serve chilled.

This sugar•free Jello with fruit is an excellent snack choice for men managing type 2 diabetes for the following reasons:

1. Sugar•free Jello is made with artificial sweeteners instead of sugar, which helps prevent blood sugar spikes.

2. The fresh or frozen fruit adds natural sweetness, fiber, and a variety of vitamins and minerals without significantly increasing the carbohydrate content.

3. The combination of the Jello and fruit creates a refreshing, hydrating, and satisfying snack.

4. This snack is easy to prepare, portable, and can be customized with different fruit combinations to provide variety.

5. The low•calorie and low•carb nature of this snack makes it a diabetes•friendly option that can be enjoyed guilt•free.

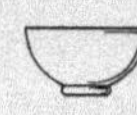 **Preparation Time : 15 min**

 **Total Time : 30 min - 1h**

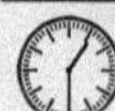 **Servings : 3-6**

Ingredients

• 1 (3 oz) package of sugar•free Jello (any flavor)
• 1 cup fresh or frozen fruit (such as berries, melon, or citrus)
• 1 cup water

Encourage the person to choose sugar•free Jello varieties and fresh or frozen fruit that are low in natural sugars, such as berries, melon, or citrus. Portion control is also important, as even sugar•free treats should be consumed in moderation as part of a balanced, diabetes•friendly diet.

Instructions

1. Preheat oven to 350°F. Line a baking sheet with parchment paper.

2. In a medium bowl, combine the rolled oats, whole wheat flour, baking soda, and salt. Mix well.

3. In a separate bowl, whisk together the unsweetened applesauce, honey, egg, and vanilla extract until well combined.

4. Gradually add the dry ingredients to the wet ingredients, mixing until just combined. Fold in the dark chocolate chips.

5. Scoop rounded tablespoons of the dough onto the prepared baking sheet, spacing them about 2 inches apart.

6. Bake for 10•12 minutes, or until the edges are lightly golden. Allow the cookies to cool on the baking sheet for 5 minutes before transferring to a wire rack to cool completely.

These cookies are a healthier alternative for men with type 2 diabetes, as they are made with whole grains, minimal added sugar, and heart•healthy dark chocolate. The oats provide fiber, and the applesauce helps keep the cookies moist without using as much oil or butter. Enjoy these cookies as a occasional treat as part of a balanced diabetes•friendly diet.

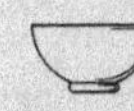 **Preparation Time : 15 min**

 **Total Time : 30 min - 1h**

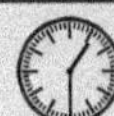 **Servings : 3-6**

Ingredients

- 1 cup rolled oats
- 1 cup whole wheat flour
- 1/2 tsp baking soda
- 1/4 tsp salt
- 1/2 cup unsweetened applesauce
- 1/4 cup honey
- 1 egg
- 1 tsp vanilla extract
- 1/2 cup dark chocolate chips (at least 70% cacao)

Instructions

1. Bring fresh, cold water to a boil in a kettle or on the stove. Remove from heat and let it cool for 2•3 minutes until the water temperature is between 160•180°F.

2. Place the green tea leaves in a teapot, infuser, or directly into a mug.

3. Pour the hot water over the tea leaves and let it steep for 1•3 minutes, depending on your desired strength. Steeping for too long can make the tea taste bitter.

4. Strain the tea leaves out if using a teapot or infuser.

5. Add honey or lemon to taste, if desired.
6. Enjoy your freshly brewed green tea!

Tips:
• Use high•quality, fresh green tea leaves for best flavor.

• Adjust the amount of tea leaves and steeping time to your personal preference.

• Avoid over•steeping the tea, as this can make it taste bitter.

• Drink green tea plain or add a touch of honey or lemon to complement the delicate flavor.

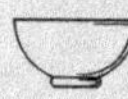 **Preparation Time : 15 min**

 **Total Time : 30 min - 1h**

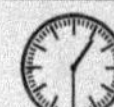 **Servings : 3-6**

Ingredients

• 1•2 teaspoons of high•quality green tea leaves
• 8 oz hot water (heated to 160•180°F)
• Optional: honey or lemon to taste

Instructions

1. In a teapot or heatproof pitcher, combine the dried chamomile flowers and lemon slices.

2. Pour the hot water over the chamomile and lemon. Stir gently to combine.

3. Allow the infusion to steep for 5•7 minutes.

4. Strain the infusion through a fine mesh sieve to remove the chamomile flowers and lemon slices.

5. Pour the infusion into cups and enjoy hot or chilled.

You can adjust the amount of chamomile and lemon to taste. Some people like to add a bit of honey as well. The chamomile provides a soothing, floral flavor while the lemon adds a bright, citrusy note. This infusion is a lovely caffeine•free herbal tea that can be enjoyed any time of day.

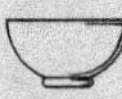 **Preparation Time : 15 min**

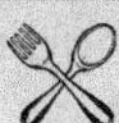 **Total Time : 30 min - 1h**

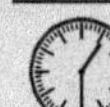 **Servings : 3-6**

Ingredients

- 2 teaspoons dried chamomile flowers
- 1 lemon, sliced
- 4 cups hot water

Instructions

1. In a large pitcher or water bottle, add the sliced lemon and fresh mint leaves.

2. Pour the 8 cups of water over the lemon and mint.

3. Refrigerate the infused water for at least 2 hours, or up to 8 hours, to allow the flavors to infuse.

4. Serve the infused water chilled, with or without ice.

5. Refill the pitcher or bottle with water as needed, reusing the lemon and mint for up to 2•3 days.

This infused water with lemon and mint is an excellent beverage choice for men managing type 2 diabetes for the following reasons:

1. Lemon is a low•glycemic fruit that won't spike blood sugar levels.

2. Mint is a refreshing, calorie•free herb that may have a positive effect on blood sugar control.

3. Infusing the water with these natural ingredients adds flavor without the need for sweeteners or other additives.

4. Staying hydrated with a low•calorie, low•carb beverage like this infused water can be beneficial for managing type 2 diabetes.

5. This homemade infused water is a cost•effective and environmentally friendly alternative to store•bought flavored waters or juices.

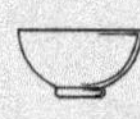 **Preparation Time : 15 min**

 **Total Time : 30 min - 1h**

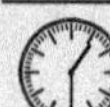 **Servings : 3-6**

Ingredients

- 1/2 cup coconut flour
- 1/4 cup unsweetened cocoa powder
- 1/4 tsp baking soda
- 1/4 tsp salt
- 3 large eggs
- 1/3 cup granulated erythritol or other zero•calorie sweetener
- 1/4 cup melted coconut oil or unsalted butter
- 1 tsp vanilla extract

Encourage the person to experiment with different fruit and herb combinations to find their favorite infused water recipes. Remind them to stay hydrated throughout the day and to avoid sugary beverages that can negatively impact blood sugar management.

Instructions

1. Add all the ingredients to a blender. Start with 1 tsp of honey and add more to taste if desired.

2. Blend on high speed until smooth and creamy, about 1 minute.

3. Pour the smoothie into a glass and enjoy immediately.

Nutrition Information (per serving):
• Calories: 200
• Total Carbs: 18g
• Fiber: 5g
• Net Carbs: 13g
• Protein: 12g
• Fat: 9g

Why this is a great smoothie for diabetes:

• Almond milk and Greek yogurt provide protein and healthy fats to help stabilize blood sugar.

• Berries are low in sugar compared to other fruits, while still providing fiber, vitamins, and antioxidants.

• Flaxseed adds fiber and healthy omega•3 fatty acids.

• Cinnamon may help improve insulin sensitivity.

• The small amount of honey provides just a touch of sweetness without spiking blood sugar too much.

This smoothie makes a nutritious, low•sugar breakfast or snack for men managing type 2 diabetes. Adjust the ingredients to your taste preferences and blood sugar needs.

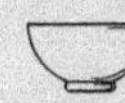 **Preparation Time : 15 min**

 **Total Time : 30 min - 1h**

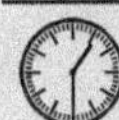 **Servings : 3-6**

Ingredients

• 1 cup unsweetened almond milk
• 1/2 cup plain Greek yogurt
• 1/2 cup frozen berries (such as raspberries, blackberries, or blueberries)
• 1 tbsp ground flaxseed
• 1 tsp cinnamon
• 1 tsp vanilla extract
• 1•2 tsp honey (optional)

Instructions

1. Wash all the vegetables and fruit thoroughly. Peel and chop them into 1•inch pieces.

2. Add the chopped carrots, cucumber, celery, beet, apple, and ginger to a juicer. Juice all the ingredients according to your juicer's instructions.

3. Once juiced, stir in the lemon juice. Taste and season with salt and pepper as desired.

4. Pour the vegetable juice into glasses and serve immediately. The juice is best consumed fresh for maximum nutrient retention.

Variations:
• Try adding other vegetables like kale, spinach, tomatoes, or parsley for extra nutrients.

• Experiment with different fruit and vegetable combinations to find your favorite flavor profile.

• For a creamier texture, you can blend the juice with a bit of yogurt or nut milk.

Enjoy your fresh, homemade vegetable juice! It's a great way to pack in lots of vitamins, minerals, and antioxidants.

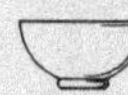 **Preparation Time : 15 min**

 **Total Time : 30 min - 1h**

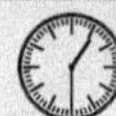 **Servings : 3-6**

Ingredients

• 2 carrots, peeled and chopped
• 1 cucumber, peeled and chopped
• 2 celery stalks, chopped
• 1 beet, peeled and chopped
• 1 apple, cored and chopped
• 1 inch piece fresh ginger, peeled
• 1 lemon, juiced
• Salt and pepper to taste

Instructions

1. Heat the almond milk in a small saucepan over medium heat, stirring frequently, until steaming hot but not boiling.

2. While the almond milk is heating, brew 1•2 shots of espresso or strong brewed coffee.

3. Pour the hot almond milk into a mug or glass.

4. Add the espresso or coffee to the almond milk.

5. If desired, stir in 1•2 teaspoons of honey or maple syrup to sweeten the latte.

6. Top with a light dusting of ground cinnamon, if desired.

7. Serve immediately and enjoy your almond milk latte!

You can adjust the ratios of almond milk to espresso/coffee to suit your taste preferences. Some people also like to froth the almond milk before adding it to the coffee for a creamier texture. This makes for a delicious, dairy•free latte option.

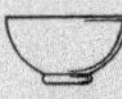 **Preparation Time : 15 min**

 **Total Time : 30 min - 1h**

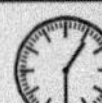 **Servings : 3-6**

Ingredients

• 1 cup unsweetened almond milk
• 1•2 shots of espresso or strong brewed coffee
• 1•2 teaspoons of honey or maple syrup (optional)
• Ground cinnamon for garnish (optional)

Instructions

1. Bring the 4 cups of water to a boil in a saucepan or kettle.

2. Remove the water from heat and add the green tea bags or loose leaf tea. Let the tea steep for 3•5 minutes.

3. Remove the tea bags or strain out the loose leaf tea. Allow the tea to cool to room temperature.

4. Once cooled, stir in 2•3 tablespoons of honey or agave nectar, if using, to sweeten the tea to your taste.

5. Fill a pitcher or glass with ice cubes. Pour the green tea over the ice.

6. Garnish with lemon slices or fresh mint leaves, if desired.

7. Refrigerate the iced green tea until ready to serve.

You can adjust the amount of tea and sweetener to your personal preferences. The iced green tea can be stored in the refrigerator for 3•4 days. Enjoy this refreshing, antioxidant•rich beverage on a hot day!

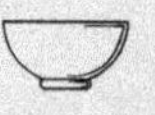 **Preparation Time : 15 min**

 **Total Time : 30 min - 1h**

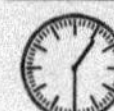 **Servings : 3-6**

Ingredients

• 4 cups water
• 4 green tea bags or 2 tablespoons loose leaf green tea
• 2•3 tablespoons honey or agave nectar (optional)
• Lemon slices or mint leaves for garnish (optional)

58. Homemade Lemonade with Stevia

Instructions

1. In a pitcher, combine the freshly squeezed lemon juice and water.

2. Add 2•3 tablespoons of liquid stevia, or to taste, depending on your desired level of sweetness. Start with 2 tablespoons and add more if needed.

3. Stir the mixture until the stevia is fully dissolved.

4. Serve the lemonade over ice, if desired.

5. Refrigerate any leftover lemonade in an airtight container for up to 5 days.

This homemade lemonade with stevia is an excellent beverage choice for men managing type 2 diabetes for the following reasons:

1. Lemons are a low•glycemic fruit, meaning they won't cause a rapid spike in blood sugar levels.

2. Stevia is a zero•calorie, natural sweetener that does not affect blood sugar, making it a great alternative to sugar or other sweeteners.

3. The combination of the tart lemon juice and the sweet stevia creates a refreshing, diabetes•friendly lemonade.

4. This homemade version allows you to control the ingredients and sweetness level, unlike store•bought lemonades that may contain added sugars.

5. Staying hydrated with a low•calorie, low•carb beverage like this lemonade can be beneficial for managing type 2 diabetes.

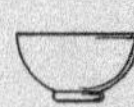 **Preparation Time : 15 min**

 **Total Time : 30 min - 1h**

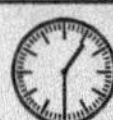 **Servings : 3-6**

Ingredients

- 6 lemons, juiced (about 3/4 cup of lemon juice)
- 4 cups water
- 2•3 tablespoons liquid stevia (or to taste)
- Ice cubes (optional)

Encourage the person to start with a smaller amount of stevia and adjust the sweetness to their personal preference. Remind them that even zero•calorie sweeteners should be consumed in moderation as part of a balanced, diabetes•friendly diet.

Instructions

1. In a large saucepan, combine the chopped tomatoes and water. Bring to a boil over medium•high heat.

2. Reduce heat to medium•low and let the tomatoes simmer for 20•25 minutes, stirring occasionally, until they have broken down and released their juices.

3. Remove the saucepan from heat and let the tomato mixture cool slightly.

4. Working in batches, carefully transfer the tomato mixture to a blender or food processor. Blend until smooth.

5. Strain the blended tomato mixture through a fine mesh sieve or cheesecloth to remove any seeds and skins. Discard the solids.

6. Stir in the salt, black pepper, and lemon juice (if using). Taste and adjust seasoning as needed.

7. Pour the tomato juice into a pitcher or jars and refrigerate until chilled, at least 2 hours.

8. Serve the tomato juice over ice. It can also be used in cocktails or other recipes that call for tomato juice.

The homemade tomato juice will keep refrigerated for 3•4 days. Enjoy this fresh, flavorful juice!

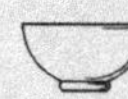 **Preparation Time : 15 min**

 **Total Time : 30 min - 1h**

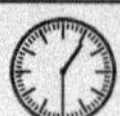 **Servings : 3-6**

Ingredients

• 3 lbs ripe tomatoes, cored and chopped
• 1/2 cup water
• 1 tsp salt
• 1/4 tsp black pepper
• 1 tbsp lemon juice (optional)

Instructions

1. Fill a glass with ice cubes.

2. Pour the chilled sparkling water over the ice.

3. Squeeze the juice from 1•2 lime wedges into the sparkling water, to taste.

4. Optionally, you can also drop the lime wedges into the glass for extra flavor and garnish.

That's it! This refreshing sparkling water with lime is a great alternative to sugary sodas or juices. The carbonation from the sparkling water provides a nice effervescence, while the lime adds a bright, citrusy flavor.

You can adjust the amount of lime to your personal taste preferences. Some people also like to add a few mint leaves or a slice of cucumber for extra flavor.

This is a versatile and hydrating beverage that can be enjoyed anytime. It's perfect for hot summer days or as a palate cleanser between meals. Enjoy!

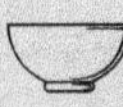 **Preparation Time : 15 min**

 **Total Time : 30 min - 1h**

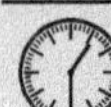 **Servings : 3-6**

Ingredients

- 1 cup chilled sparkling water
- 1•2 lime wedges

Instructions

1. Fill a medium saucepan with about 1 inch of water and bring it to a boil over high heat.

2. Add the broccoli florets to a steamer basket and place the basket in the saucepan. Cover and steam the broccoli for 5•7 minutes, until tender•crisp.

3. Carefully remove the steamer basket from the saucepan. Transfer the steamed broccoli to a serving bowl.

4. Drizzle the lemon juice and olive oil over the broccoli. Sprinkle with salt and black pepper.

5. Toss gently to coat the broccoli evenly with the lemon, oil, salt, and pepper.

6. Serve the steamed broccoli warm or at room temperature.

This dish is a great option for men with type 2 diabetes for a few reasons:

• Broccoli is high in fiber, which can help regulate blood sugar levels.

• Lemon juice provides a bright, tangy flavor without adding any sugar.

• The olive oil contains healthy monounsaturated fats that can help improve insulin sensitivity.

• It's a simple, low•calorie side dish that pairs well with lean proteins.

Enjoy this easy and nutritious steamed broccoli with lemon!

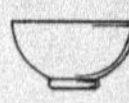 **Preparation Time : 15 min**

 **Total Time : 30 min - 1h**

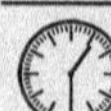 **Servings : 3-6**

Ingredients

• 1 lb broccoli florets
• 2 tbsp fresh lemon juice
• 1 tsp olive oil
• 1/4 tsp salt
• 1/8 tsp black pepper

Instructions

1. In a large skillet or wok, heat the olive oil over medium heat. Add the minced garlic and red pepper flakes (if using) and cook for 1 minute, stirring constantly, until fragrant.

2. Add the spinach to the skillet in batches, stirring constantly, until the spinach is wilted down, about 2•3 minutes per batch.

3. Once all the spinach is wilted, season with salt and pepper to taste.

4. Serve the garlic sautéed spinach warm, as a side dish. Enjoy!

The key is to sauté the garlic briefly before adding the spinach to infuse the oil with the garlic flavor. The spinach cooks down quickly, so it's important to work in batches to avoid overcrowding the pan. This simple preparation allows the fresh spinach flavor to shine.

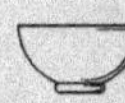 **Preparation Time : 15 min**

 **Total Time : 30 min - 1h**

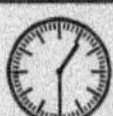 **Servings : 3-6**

Ingredients

- 1 lb fresh spinach, washed and stems removed
- 2 tbsp olive oil
- 3 cloves garlic, minced
- 1/4 tsp red pepper flakes (optional)
- Salt and pepper to taste

Instructions

1. Preheat your oven to 400°F (200°C). Line a large baking sheet with parchment paper.

2. In a large bowl, toss the cauliflower florets with the olive oil, garlic powder, paprika, salt, and black pepper until the cauliflower is evenly coated.

3. Spread the seasoned cauliflower in a single layer on the prepared baking sheet.

4. Roast the cauliflower for 20•25 minutes, flipping halfway through, until it is tender and lightly browned on the edges.

5. Remove the roasted cauliflower from the oven and serve hot.

This roasted cauliflower dish is a great option for men managing type 2 diabetes for a few reasons:

• Cauliflower is low in carbs and high in fiber, which can help regulate blood sugar levels.

• The healthy fats from the olive oil can improve insulin sensitivity.

• The simple seasoning adds flavor without any added sugars.

• Roasting brings out the natural sweetness of the cauliflower.

You can serve the roasted cauliflower as a side dish or incorporate it into other meals, such as salads or grain bowls. It's a versatile and nutritious option that can be enjoyed by everyone, including those with type 2 diabetes.

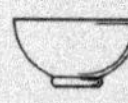 **Preparation Time : 15 min**

 **Total Time : 30 min - 1h**

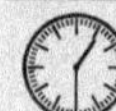 **Servings : 3-6**

Ingredients

• 1 head of cauliflower, cut into florets
• 2 tbsp olive oil
• 1 tsp garlic powder
• 1 tsp paprika
• 1/2 tsp salt
• 1/4 tsp black pepper

Instructions

1. In a medium saucepan, combine the rinsed quinoa and broth. Bring to a boil over high heat.

2. Once boiling, reduce heat to low, cover, and simmer for 15•20 minutes, until the quinoa is tender and the liquid is absorbed.

3. In a large skillet, heat the olive oil over medium heat. Add the onion and sauté for 3•4 minutes until translucent.

4. Add the garlic, bell peppers, and zucchini/squash. Sauté for 5•7 minutes, until the vegetables are tender.

5. Fluff the cooked quinoa with a fork and add it to the vegetable mixture.

6. Stir in the thyme, cumin, salt, and black pepper. Cook for 2•3 minutes to allow the flavors to blend.

7. Remove from heat and stir in the chopped parsley, if using. Serve the quinoa pilaf warm.

This quinoa pilaf is a great option for men with type 2 diabetes for a few reasons:

• Quinoa is a whole grain that is high in fiber and protein, which can help regulate blood sugar levels.

• The vegetables add nutrients, fiber, and minimal carbs.

• The simple seasoning provides flavor without added sugars.

• It's a filling and satisfying dish that can be enjoyed as a main course or side.

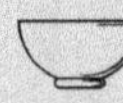 **Preparation Time : 15 min**

 **Total Time : 30 min - 1h**

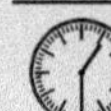 **Servings : 3-6**

Ingredients

• 1 cup uncooked quinoa, rinsed
• 2 cups low•sodium vegetable or chicken broth
• 1 tbsp olive oil
• 1 onion, diced
• 2 garlic cloves, minced
• 1 cup diced bell peppers (any color)
• 1 cup diced zucchini or yellow squash
• 1 tsp dried thyme
• 1/2 tsp ground cumin
• 1/4 tsp salt
• 1/4 tsp black pepper
• 2 tbsp chopped fresh parsley (optional)

Instructions

1. Preheat your grill or grill pan to medium•high heat.

2. In a large bowl, toss the asparagus spears with the olive oil, lemon zest, lemon juice, garlic powder, salt, and black pepper until the asparagus is evenly coated.

3. Arrange the seasoned asparagus in a single layer on the preheated grill or grill pan.

4. Grill the asparagus for 5•7 minutes, turning occasionally, until tender•crisp and lightly charred.

5. Remove the grilled asparagus from the heat and serve immediately.

This grilled asparagus dish is a great option for men managing type 2 diabetes for a few reasons:

• Asparagus is low in carbs and high in fiber, which can help regulate blood sugar levels.

• The healthy fats from the olive oil can improve insulin sensitivity.

• The lemon and garlic add flavor without any added sugars.

• Grilling brings out the natural sweetness of the asparagus while adding a delicious smoky flavor.

You can serve the grilled asparagus as a side dish or incorporate it into other meals, such as salads or grain bowls. It's a versatile and nutritious option that can be enjoyed by everyone, including those with type 2 diabetes.

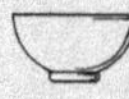 **Preparation Time : 15 min**

 **Total Time : 30 min - 1h**

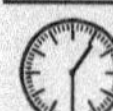 **Servings : 3-6**

Ingredients

• 1 lb asparagus, woody ends trimmed
• 2 tbsp olive oil
• 1 tsp lemon zest
• 1 tbsp lemon juice
• 1/2 tsp garlic powder
• 1/4 tsp salt
• 1/4 tsp black pepper

Instructions

1. In a large bowl, combine the sliced cucumbers and red onion.

2. In a small bowl, whisk together the apple cider vinegar, olive oil, Dijon mustard, honey (if using), salt, and black pepper.

3. Pour the vinegar dressing over the cucumber and onion mixture. Toss gently to coat.

4. Cover the bowl and refrigerate the cucumber salad for at least 30 minutes, or up to 2 hours, to allow the flavors to meld.

5. Just before serving, stir in the chopped fresh dill, if using.

This cucumber salad is a great option for men managing type 2 diabetes for a few reasons:

• Cucumbers are low in carbs and high in water content, which can help hydrate the body and regulate blood sugar levels.

• The apple cider vinegar may help improve insulin sensitivity and lower blood sugar levels.

• The small amount of honey (if using) provides a touch of sweetness without a significant impact on blood sugar.

• The healthy fats from the olive oil can also help improve insulin sensitivity.

This refreshing and flavorful cucumber salad can be served as a side dish or enjoyed as a light snack. It's a versatile and nutritious option that can be part of a balanced diet for those with type 2 diabetes.

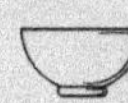 **Preparation Time : 15 min**

 **Total Time : 30 min - 1h**

 **Servings : 3-6**

Ingredients

• 2 medium cucumbers, thinly sliced
• 1/2 red onion, thinly sliced
• 2 tbsp apple cider vinegar
• 1 tbsp olive oil
• 1 tsp Dijon mustard
• 1 tsp honey (optional)
• 1/4 tsp salt
• 1/4 tsp black pepper
• 2 tbsp chopped fresh dill (optional)

Instructions

1. Preheat your oven to 400°F (200°C). Line a large baking sheet with parchment paper.

2. In a large bowl, toss the sweet potato fries with the olive oil, paprika, garlic powder, salt, and black pepper until the fries are evenly coated.

3. Spread the seasoned sweet potato fries in a single layer on the prepared baking sheet, making sure they are not touching each other.

4. Bake for 20•25 minutes, flipping the fries halfway through, until they are crispy and lightly browned on the edges.

5. Remove the baked sweet potato fries from the oven and serve hot.

Tips:
• For crispier fries, you can soak the cut sweet potatoes in cold water for 30 minutes before patting them dry and tossing with the seasonings.

• Try adding other spices like chili powder, cumin, or cayenne pepper for different flavor variations.

• Serve the sweet potato fries with your favorite dipping sauce, such as ranch, honey mustard, or barbecue sauce.

Sweet potato fries are a healthier alternative to regular french fries, as they are packed with vitamins, minerals, and fiber. Enjoy this easy and delicious side dish!

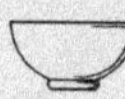 **Preparation Time : 15 min**

 **Total Time : 30 min - 1h**

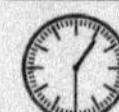 **Servings : 3-6**

Ingredients

• 2 lbs sweet potatoes, peeled and cut into 1/2•inch thick fry shapes
• 2 tbsp olive oil
• 1 tsp paprika
• 1/2 tsp garlic powder
• 1/2 tsp salt
• 1/4 tsp black pepper

Instructions

1. Wash and dry the cauliflower florets thoroughly.

2. Working in batches, place the cauliflower florets in a food processor and pulse until the cauliflower is broken down into small, rice•like pieces. Be careful not to over•process, as you don't want the cauliflower to become a puree.

Alternatively, you can grate the cauliflower florets using a box grater to create the "rice" texture.

3. (Optional) In a large skillet, heat the olive oil over medium heat. Add the riced cauliflower and sauté for 3•5 minutes, stirring occasionally, until the cauliflower is tender and lightly browned.

4. Season the cauliflower rice with salt and pepper to taste.

That's it! Your homemade cauliflower rice is now ready to use.

Some ways to use cauliflower rice:
• As a low•carb substitute for regular rice in dishes like stir•fries, burrito bowls, or fried rice.
• As a base for grain bowls or salads.
• Sautéed with vegetables and seasonings as a side dish.
• Baked into casseroles or used in stuffed peppers or tomatoes.

Cauliflower rice is a great option for those looking to reduce their carb intake, as it's low in carbs and high in fiber, vitamins, and minerals. Enjoy this versatile and healthy alternative to traditional rice!

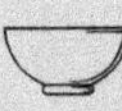 **Preparation Time : 15 min**

 **Total Time : 30 min - 1h**

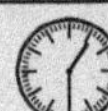 **Servings : 3-6**

Ingredients

• 1 medium head of cauliflower, cut into florets
• 1 tbsp olive oil (optional)
• Salt and pepper to taste

Instructions

1. Preheat your oven to 400°F (200°C). Line a baking sheet with parchment paper.

2. In a large bowl, toss the trimmed and halved Brussels sprouts with the olive oil, salt, and black pepper until the sprouts are evenly coated.

3. Spread the seasoned Brussels sprouts in a single layer on the prepared baking sheet.

4. Roast the Brussels sprouts for 18•22 minutes, tossing halfway, until they are tender and lightly browned.

5. In a small saucepan, combine the balsamic vinegar and honey. Bring the mixture to a simmer over medium heat, stirring occasionally, until it thickens into a glaze, about 3•5 minutes.

6. Remove the roasted Brussels sprouts from the oven and drizzle the balsamic glaze over the top, tossing gently to coat.

7. Serve the Brussels sprouts with balsamic glaze immediately.

This Brussels sprouts dish is a great option for men managing type 2 diabetes for a few reasons:

• Brussels sprouts are low in carbs and high in fiber, which can help regulate blood sugar levels.
• The balsamic vinegar may help improve insulin sensitivity and lower blood sugar levels.
• The small amount of honey provides a touch of sweetness without a significant impact on blood sugar.
• The dish is simple, flavorful, and can be easily incorporated into a balanced, diabetes•friendly meal.

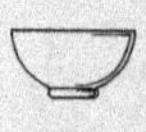 **Preparation Time : 15 min**

 **Total Time : 30 min - 1h**

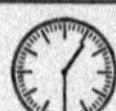 **Servings : 3-6**

Ingredients

• 1 lb Brussels sprouts, trimmed and halved
• 2 tbsp olive oil
• 1/4 tsp salt
• 1/8 tsp black pepper
• 2 tbsp balsamic vinegar
• 1 tbsp honey

Instructions

1. Place the cubed butternut squash in a large pot and cover with water. Bring to a boil over high heat.

2. Reduce the heat to medium•low and simmer the squash for 15•20 minutes, until very tender when pierced with a fork.

3. Drain the cooked squash in a colander and return it to the pot.

4. Add the butter, milk, cinnamon, nutmeg, salt, and pepper to the pot. Mash the squash with a potato masher or an electric hand mixer until smooth and creamy.

5. Taste and adjust seasoning as needed, adding more salt, pepper, or spices to your preference.

6. Serve the mashed butternut squash warm.

This mashed butternut squash makes a delicious and nutritious side dish. Butternut squash is high in fiber, vitamins, and minerals, making it a great option for those managing type 2 diabetes.

The cinnamon and nutmeg add warmth and depth of flavor, while the butter and milk (or non•dairy milk) provide a creamy texture. This dish is naturally sweet, so there's no need for added sugars.

Enjoy this easy and comforting mashed butternut squash alongside roasted meats, grilled fish, or as part of a fall•inspired meal.

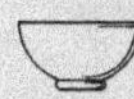 **Preparation Time : 15 min**

 **Total Time : 30 min - 1h**

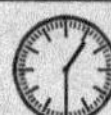 **Servings : 3-6**

Ingredients

• 1 medium butternut squash, peeled, seeded, and cubed (about 4 cups cubed)
• 2 tbsp unsalted butter
• 1/4 cup milk or unsweetened almond milk
• 1/2 tsp ground cinnamon
• 1/4 tsp ground nutmeg
• 1/4 tsp salt
• 1/8 tsp black pepper

Instructions

1. In a large saucepan or Dutch oven, heat the olive oil over medium heat. Add the diced onion and sauté for 5•7 minutes until translucent.

2. Add the minced garlic and sauté for an additional 1•2 minutes until fragrant.

3. Pour in the can of diced tomatoes, including the juices, and the vegetable or chicken broth. Stir to combine.

4. Add the dried basil, dried oregano, red pepper flakes (if using), salt, and black pepper. Bring the soup to a simmer.

5. Reduce the heat to low and let the soup simmer for 15•20 minutes, stirring occasionally, to allow the flavors to meld.

6. Remove the soup from heat and stir in the chopped fresh basil.

7. Using an immersion blender or carefully transferring the soup to a blender, puree the soup until smooth and creamy.

8. Taste and adjust seasoning as needed.

9. Serve the tomato basil soup hot, garnished with additional fresh basil if desired.

This tomato basil soup is a great option for men managing type 2 diabetes for a few reasons:

Enjoy this delicious and nutritious tomato basil soup!

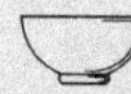 **Preparation Time : 15 min**

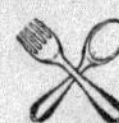 **Total Time : 30 min - 1h**

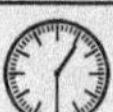 **Servings : 3-6**

Ingredients

• 2 tbsp olive oil
• 1 onion, diced
• 3 garlic cloves, minced
• 1 (28 oz) can diced tomatoes
• 2 cups low•sodium vegetable or chicken broth
• 1 tsp dried basil
• 1/2 tsp dried oregano
• 1/4 tsp red pepper flakes (optional)
• 1/4 tsp salt
• 1/8 tsp black pepper
• 1/4 cup fresh basil leaves, chopped

• Tomatoes are low in carbs and high in antioxidants, which can help regulate blood sugar levels.

• The fresh and dried herbs add flavor without any added sugars.

• The olive oil provides healthy fats that can improve insulin sensitivity.

• It's a comforting and satisfying soup that can be easily incorporated into a balanced, diabetes•friendly diet.

Instructions

1. In a large pot or Dutch oven, heat the olive oil over medium heat. Add the onion, carrots, celery, and garlic. Sauté for 5•7 minutes until the vegetables are softened.

2. Add the chicken pieces to the pot and cook for 3•4 minutes, stirring occasionally, until the chicken is lightly browned.

3. Pour in the chicken broth and add the diced tomatoes, kale/spinach, thyme, oregano, salt, pepper, and bay leaves. Stir to combine.

4. Bring the soup to a boil, then reduce the heat and let it simmer for 15 minutes.

5. Add the uncooked pasta to the pot and continue simmering for 10•12 minutes, or until the pasta is tender.

6. Remove the bay leaves before serving.

7. Ladle the chicken and vegetable soup into bowls and enjoy!

This hearty soup is a great option for those managing type 2 diabetes. It's packed with lean protein from the chicken, fiber•rich vegetables, and whole grain pasta. The simple seasoning provides flavor without added sugars. Enjoy this comforting and nutritious soup!

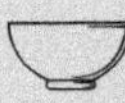 **Preparation Time : 15 min**

 **Total Time : 30 min - 1h**

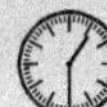 **Servings : 3-6**

Ingredients

- 2 tbsp olive oil
- 1 onion, diced
- 3 carrots, peeled and sliced
- 3 celery stalks, sliced
- 3 garlic cloves, minced
- 1 lb boneless, skinless chicken breasts, cut into 1•inch pieces
- 6 cups low•sodium chicken broth
- 1 (15 oz) can diced tomatoes
- 2 cups chopped kale or spinach
- 1 tsp dried thyme
- 1 tsp dried oregano
- 1/2 tsp salt
- 1/4 tsp black pepper
- 2 bay leaves
- 1 cup uncooked whole wheat pasta (such as elbow macaroni or ditalini)

Instructions

1. In a large pot or Dutch oven, heat the olive oil over medium heat. Add the onion, carrots, celery and garlic. Sauté for 5•7 minutes until the vegetables are softened.

2. Stir in the oregano, basil and red pepper flakes (if using). Cook for 1 minute until fragrant.

3. Add the diced tomatoes, broth, kidney beans, and cannellini beans. Bring the soup to a boil.

4. Reduce heat and let the soup simmer for 15 minutes.

5. Stir in the kale/spinach and pasta. Cook for 8•10 minutes more until the pasta is tender.

6. Season with salt and pepper to taste.

7. Serve the minestrone soup hot, topped with grated Parmesan cheese if desired.

This hearty minestrone is packed with vegetables, beans, and whole grains for a nutritious and filling meal. It's perfect for a cozy dinner on a chilly day. Enjoy!

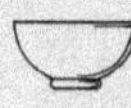 **Preparation Time : 15 min**

 **Total Time : 30 min - 1h**

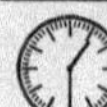 **Servings : 3-6**

Ingredients

- 2 tbsp olive oil
- 1 onion, diced
- 3 carrots, peeled and diced
- 3 celery stalks, diced
- 4 garlic cloves, minced
- 1 tsp dried oregano
- 1 tsp dried basil
- 1/4 tsp red pepper flakes (optional)
- 1 (28 oz) can diced tomatoes
- 4 cups vegetable or chicken broth
- 1 (15 oz) can kidney beans, drained and rinsed
- 1 (15 oz) can cannellini beans, drained and rinsed
- 2 cups chopped kale or spinach
- 1 cup small pasta (like ditalini or elbow macaroni)
- Salt and pepper to taste
- Grated Parmesan cheese for serving (optional)

Instructions

1. In a large saucepan or Dutch oven, heat the olive oil over medium heat. Add the diced onion and sauté for 5•7 minutes until translucent.

2. Add the minced garlic and sauté for an additional 1•2 minutes until fragrant.

3. Stir in the pumpkin puree, chicken or vegetable broth, cinnamon, ginger, nutmeg, salt, and black pepper. Bring the soup to a simmer.

4. Reduce the heat to low and let the soup simmer for 15•20 minutes, stirring occasionally, to allow the flavors to meld.

5. Remove the soup from heat and stir in the unsweetened almond milk (or low•fat milk).

6. Using an immersion blender or carefully transferring the soup to a blender, puree the soup until smooth and creamy.

7. Taste and adjust seasoning as needed.

8. Serve the pumpkin soup hot, garnished with chopped fresh parsley if desired.

This pumpkin soup is a great option for men managing type 2 diabetes for a few reasons:

• Pumpkin is low in carbs and high in fiber, vitamins, and antioxidants, which can help regulate blood sugar levels.
• The simple seasoning provides flavor without added sugars.
• The use of almond milk or low•fat milk keeps the soup creamy without adding too much fat.
• It's a comforting and satisfying soup that can be easily incorporated into a balanced, diabetes•friendly diet.

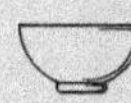 **Preparation Time : 15 min**

 **Total Time : 30 min - 1h**

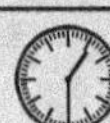 **Servings : 3-6**

Ingredients

• 1 tbsp olive oil
• 1 onion, diced
• 3 garlic cloves, minced
• 1 (15 oz) can pumpkin puree
• 4 cups low•sodium chicken or vegetable broth
• 1 tsp ground cinnamon
• 1/2 tsp ground ginger
• 1/4 tsp ground nutmeg
• 1/4 tsp salt
• 1/8 tsp black pepper
• 1/4 cup unsweetened almond milk (or low•fat milk)
• 2 tbsp chopped fresh parsley (optional)

Instructions

1. In a large pot or Dutch oven, heat the olive oil over medium heat. Add the diced onion and sauté for 5•7 minutes until translucent.

2. Add the minced garlic and sauté for 1 minute until fragrant.

3. Stir in the rinsed lentils, vegetable or chicken broth, and diced tomatoes (with their juices). Bring the soup to a boil.

4. Reduce the heat to medium•low and let the soup simmer for 20•25 minutes, or until the lentils are tender.

5. Stir in the chopped fresh spinach, cumin, oregano, red pepper flakes (if using), salt, and black pepper. Cook for an additional 5 minutes, until the spinach is wilted.

6. Taste and adjust seasoning as needed.

7. Serve the lentil and spinach soup hot.

This lentil and spinach soup is an excellent option for men managing type 2 diabetes for several reasons:

• Lentils are high in fiber and protein, which can help regulate blood sugar levels.

• Spinach is low in carbs and packed with vitamins, minerals, and antioxidants.

• The simple seasoning provides flavor without added sugars.

• The soup is filling and nutritious, making it a great option for a main course or hearty side dish

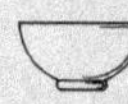 **Preparation Time : 15 min**

 **Total Time : 30 min - 1h**

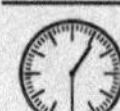 **Servings : 3-6**

Ingredients

• 1 tbsp olive oil
• 1 onion, diced
• 3 garlic cloves, minced
• 1 cup dried brown or green lentils, rinsed
• 4 cups low•sodium vegetable or chicken broth
• 1 (14.5 oz) can diced tomatoes
• 2 cups chopped fresh spinach
• 1 tsp ground cumin
• 1/2 tsp dried oregano
• 1/4 tsp red pepper flakes (optional)
• 1/2 tsp salt
• 1/4 tsp black pepper

You can customize the soup by adding other vegetables, such as carrots or celery, or by using different types of lentils. Enjoy this delicious and diabetes•friendly lentil and spinach soup!

Instructions

1. In a large saucepan, bring the broth to a boil over medium•high heat. Add the chopped broccoli, onion, and garlic. Reduce heat to medium•low and simmer for 10•12 minutes, until the broccoli is tender.

2. In a small bowl, whisk together the flour and milk until smooth. Slowly pour the milk mixture into the saucepan, whisking constantly, to thicken the soup.

3. Reduce heat to low and stir in the shredded low•fat cheddar cheese, ground mustard, cayenne pepper (if using), salt, and black pepper. Cook, stirring frequently, until the cheese is melted and the soup is heated through, about 5 minutes.

4. Carefully use an immersion blender to partially puree the soup, leaving some broccoli pieces intact. Alternatively, you can transfer about half the soup to a blender, blend until smooth, then return it to the saucepan.

5. Taste and adjust seasoning as needed. Serve the broccoli cheddar soup hot.

This low•fat broccoli cheddar soup is a great option for men managing type 2 diabetes for a few reasons:

• Broccoli is low in carbs and high in fiber, vitamins, and minerals.
• The use of low•fat milk and cheese reduces the overall fat and calorie content.
• The simple seasoning provides flavor without added sugars.
• It's a comforting and satisfying soup that can be easily incorporated into a balanced, diabetes•friendly diet.

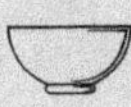 **Preparation Time : 15 min**

 **Total Time : 30 min - 1h**

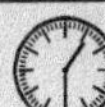 **Servings : 3-6**

Ingredients

• 2 cups low•sodium chicken or vegetable broth
• 3 cups chopped broccoli florets
• 1 medium onion, diced
• 2 garlic cloves, minced
• 2 tbsp all•purpose flour
• 1 cup low•fat milk
• 3/4 cup shredded low•fat cheddar cheese
• 1/4 tsp ground mustard
• 1/4 tsp cayenne pepper (optional)
• 1/4 tsp salt
• 1/8 tsp black pepper

77. Zucchini and Basil Soup

Instructions

1. In a large pot or Dutch oven, heat the olive oil over medium heat. Add the diced onion and sauté for 5•7 minutes until translucent.

2. Add the minced garlic and sauté for 1•2 minutes until fragrant.

3. Stir in the diced zucchini and chicken or vegetable broth. Bring the soup to a boil.

4. Reduce the heat to medium•low and let the soup simmer for 15•20 minutes, or until the zucchini is very tender.

5. Remove the pot from heat and stir in the chopped fresh basil, lemon juice, salt, and black pepper.

6. Using an immersion blender or carefully transferring the soup to a blender, puree the soup until smooth and creamy.

7. Taste and adjust seasoning as needed.

8. Serve the zucchini and basil soup warm, garnished with a sprinkle of grated Parmesan cheese (if using).

This nourishing soup can be enjoyed as a starter or a light main course. Pair it with a fresh salad or a piece of grilled protein for a complete, diabetes•friendly meal.

Enjoy this delicious and healthy zucchini and basil soup!

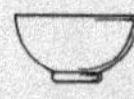 **Preparation Time : 15 min**

 **Total Time : 30 min - 1h**

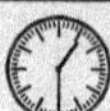 **Servings : 3-6**

Ingredients

• 2 tbsp olive oil
• 1 onion, diced
• 3 garlic cloves, minced
• 3 medium zucchini, diced
• 4 cups low•sodium chicken or vegetable broth
• 1/2 cup fresh basil leaves, chopped
• 1 tsp lemon juice
• 1/2 tsp salt
• 1/4 tsp black pepper
• 2 tbsp grated Parmesan cheese (optional)

This zucchini and basil soup is an excellent option for men managing type 2 diabetes for several reasons:

• Zucchini is low in carbs and high in fiber, vitamins, and minerals.

• Fresh basil provides a bright, herbal flavor without any added sugars.

• The lemon juice adds a refreshing tanginess.

• The soup is creamy and satisfying, yet low in calories and fat.

Instructions

1. In a large pot or Dutch oven, heat the olive oil over medium•high heat. Add the beef cubes and brown on all sides, about 5•7 minutes total. Remove the beef from the pot and set aside.

2. Reduce the heat to medium and add the diced onion, sliced carrots, and sliced celery to the pot. Sauté for 5•7 minutes until the vegetables are softened.

3. Add the minced garlic and sauté for 1•2 minutes until fragrant.

4. Pour in the beef or chicken broth and stir in the rinsed pearl barley, diced tomatoes, dried thyme, dried rosemary, salt, and black pepper.

5. Bring the soup to a boil, then reduce the heat to medium•low. Simmer for 30•40 minutes, or until the barley is tender.

6. Add the browned beef back to the pot and continue simmering for an additional 10•15 minutes.

7. If using, stir in the chopped kale or spinach during the last 5 minutes of cooking.

8. Taste and adjust seasoning as needed.

9. Serve the beef and barley soup hot.

This hearty and nourishing soup can be enjoyed as a main course or paired with a fresh salad for a complete, diabetes•friendly meal.

Enjoy this delicious beef and barley soup!

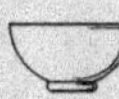 **Preparation Time : 15 min**

 **Total Time : 30 min - 1h**

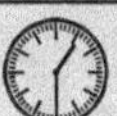 **Servings : 3-6**

Ingredients

• 1 lb lean beef stew meat, cut into 1•inch cubes
• 2 tbsp olive oil
• 1 onion, diced
• 3 carrots, peeled and sliced
• 3 celery stalks, sliced
• 4 garlic cloves, minced
• 6 cups low•sodium beef or chicken broth
• 1 cup pearl barley, rinsed
• 1 (14.5 oz) can diced tomatoes
• 2 tsp dried thyme
• 1 tsp dried rosemary
• 1/2 tsp salt
• 1/4 tsp black pepper
• 2 cups chopped kale or spinach (optional)

This beef and barley soup is a great option for men managing type 2 diabetes for several reasons:

• Lean beef provides protein to help stabilize blood sugar levels.
• Barley is a whole grain that is high in fiber, which can help regulate blood sugar.
• The vegetables add nutrients and minimal carbs.
• The simple seasoning provides flavor without added sugars.

Instructions

1. In a large pot or Dutch oven, heat the olive oil over medium heat. Add the diced onion and sauté for 5•7 minutes until translucent.

2. Add the minced garlic and grated ginger. Cook for 1•2 minutes, stirring constantly, until fragrant.

3. Add the sliced carrots, chicken or vegetable broth, cumin, coriander, cayenne (if using), salt, and black pepper. Stir to combine.

4. Bring the soup to a boil, then reduce the heat and let it simmer for 20•25 minutes, or until the carrots are very tender.

5. Using an immersion blender or carefully transferring the soup to a blender, puree the soup until smooth and creamy.

6. Taste and adjust seasoning as needed.

7. Serve the carrot and ginger soup warm, topped with a dollop of plain Greek yogurt and chopped fresh cilantro, if desired.

This nourishing soup can be enjoyed as a starter or a light main course. Pair it with a fresh salad or a piece of grilled protein for a complete, diabetes•friendly meal.

Enjoy this delicious and healthy carrot and ginger soup!

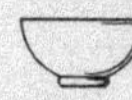 **Preparation Time : 15 min**

 **Total Time : 30 min - 1h**

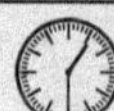 **Servings : 3-6**

Ingredients

• 2 tbsp olive oil
• 1 onion, diced
• 3 cloves garlic, minced
• 1 tbsp grated fresh ginger
• 1 lb carrots, peeled and sliced
• 4 cups low•sodium chicken or vegetable broth
• 1 tsp ground cumin
• 1/2 tsp ground coriander
• 1/4 tsp cayenne pepper (optional)
• 1/2 tsp salt
• 1/4 tsp black pepper
• 2 tbsp plain Greek yogurt (optional, for serving)
• Chopped fresh cilantro (optional, for serving)

This carrot and ginger soup is an excellent option for men managing type 2 diabetes for a few reasons:

• Carrots are low in carbs and high in fiber, vitamins, and antioxidants.
• Ginger may help improve insulin sensitivity and reduce inflammation.
• The simple seasoning provides flavor without added sugars.
• The Greek yogurt topping adds a creamy texture and protein.

Instructions

1. In a large pot or Dutch oven, heat the olive oil over medium heat. Add the diced onion and sauté for 5•7 minutes until translucent.

2. Add the minced garlic, cumin, oregano, and cayenne (if using). Cook for 1•2 minutes, stirring constantly, until fragrant.

3. Stir in the rinsed and drained black beans, vegetable or chicken broth, diced tomatoes, and bay leaf. Bring the soup to a boil.

4. Reduce the heat to medium•low and let the soup simmer for 20•25 minutes, stirring occasionally, until slightly thickened.

5. Remove the bay leaf. Use an immersion blender or transfer about half the soup to a blender and puree until smooth. Return the pureed soup to the pot.

6. Stir in the salt and black pepper. Taste and adjust seasoning as needed.

7. Serve the black bean soup hot, garnished with chopped cilantro and accompanied by lime wedges, if desired.

This black bean soup is a great option for those managing type 2 diabetes for a few reasons:

• Black beans are high in fiber and protein, which can help regulate blood sugar levels.
• The simple seasoning provides flavor without added sugars.
• The soup is filling and nutritious, making it a great option for a main course or hearty side dish.

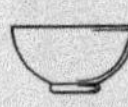 **Preparation Time : 15 min**

 **Total Time : 30 min - 1h**

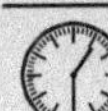 **Servings : 3-6**

Ingredients

• 2 tbsp olive oil
• 1 onion, diced
• 3 garlic cloves, minced
• 2 tsp ground cumin
• 1 tsp dried oregano
• 1/4 tsp cayenne pepper (optional)
• 2 (15 oz) cans black beans, rinsed and drained
• 4 cups low•sodium vegetable or chicken broth
• 1 (14.5 oz) can diced tomatoes
• 1 bay leaf
• 1/2 tsp salt
• 1/4 tsp black pepper
• Chopped cilantro for garnish (optional)
• Lime wedges for serving (optional)

You can customize the soup by adding other vegetables, such as bell peppers or carrots, or by using different types of beans. Enjoy this delicious and diabetes•friendly black bean soup!

Instructions

1. In a large salad bowl, combine the baby spinach leaves, sliced strawberries, sliced almonds, and crumbled feta cheese.

2. In a small bowl, whisk together the balsamic vinegar, olive oil, Dijon mustard, honey (if using), salt, and black pepper to make the dressing.

3. Drizzle the dressing over the salad and toss gently to coat the ingredients evenly.

4. Serve the spinach and strawberry salad immediately.

This salad is a great option for men managing type 2 diabetes for several reasons:

• Spinach is low in carbs and high in fiber, vitamins, and minerals.

• Strawberries are a low•glycemic fruit that can help regulate blood sugar levels.

• The healthy fats from the olive oil and almonds can improve insulin sensitivity.

• The small amount of honey (if using) provides a touch of sweetness without a significant impact on blood sugar.

• The simple balsamic vinaigrette dressing adds flavor without added sugars.

This refreshing and nutritious salad can be enjoyed as a light main course or a side dish. It's a versatile option that can be easily incorporated into a balanced, diabetes•friendly diet.

Enjoy this delicious spinach and strawberry salad!

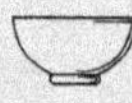
Preparation Time : 15 min

Total Time : 30 min - 1h

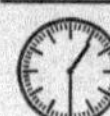
Servings : 3-6

Ingredients

• 5 oz baby spinach leaves
• 1 cup fresh strawberries, sliced
• 1/4 cup sliced almonds
• 2 tbsp crumbled feta cheese
• 2 tbsp balsamic vinegar
• 1 tbsp olive oil
• 1 tsp Dijon mustard
• 1 tsp honey (optional)
• 1/4 tsp salt
• 1/8 tsp black pepper

Instructions

1. In a medium saucepan, combine the rinsed quinoa and broth. Bring to a boil over high heat.

2. Once boiling, reduce heat to low, cover, and simmer for 15•20 minutes, until the quinoa is tender and the liquid is absorbed.

3. Transfer the cooked quinoa to a large bowl and let it cool slightly.

4. Add the chopped kale, cherry tomatoes, crumbled feta, and sliced almonds to the bowl with the quinoa.

5. In a small bowl, whisk together the olive oil, lemon juice, Dijon mustard, minced garlic, salt, and black pepper.

6. Pour the dressing over the salad and toss gently to coat.

7. Serve the kale and quinoa salad immediately or refrigerate until ready to serve.

This kale and quinoa salad is a great option for men managing type 2 diabetes for several reasons:

• Quinoa is a whole grain that is high in fiber and protein, which can help regulate blood sugar levels.

• Kale is low in carbs and high in vitamins, minerals, and antioxidants.

• The cherry tomatoes, feta, and almonds provide additional nutrients and healthy fats.

• The simple lemon•Dijon dressing adds flavor without any added sugars

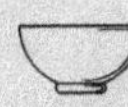 **Preparation Time : 15 min**

 **Total Time : 30 min - 1h**

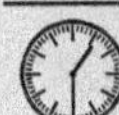 **Servings : 3-6**

Ingredients

• 1 cup uncooked quinoa, rinsed
• 2 cups low•sodium vegetable or chicken broth
• 1 bunch kale, stems removed and leaves chopped
• 1 cup cherry tomatoes, halved
• 1/2 cup crumbled feta cheese
• 1/4 cup sliced almonds
• 2 tbsp olive oil
• 2 tbsp lemon juice
• 1 tsp Dijon mustard
• 1 garlic clove, minced
• 1/4 tsp salt
• 1/8 tsp black pepper

This salad is a nutritious and filling meal that can be enjoyed on its own or paired with grilled chicken or fish for a complete, diabetes•friendly lunch or dinner.

Enjoy this delicious and diabetes•friendly kale and quinoa salad!

Instructions

1. In a large bowl, combine the shredded green cabbage, shredded red cabbage, grated carrot, and julienned apple.

2. In a small bowl, whisk together the apple cider vinegar, olive oil, Dijon mustard, honey (if using), salt, and black pepper to make the dressing.

3. Pour the dressing over the cabbage and vegetable mixture and toss gently to coat everything evenly.

4. Cover the slaw and refrigerate for at least 30 minutes, or up to 2 hours, to allow the flavors to meld.

5. Just before serving, stir in the chopped fresh parsley, if using.

This cabbage slaw is a great option for men managing type 2 diabetes for several reasons:

• Cabbage and carrots are low in carbs and high in fiber, vitamins, and minerals.

• Apples add a touch of natural sweetness without a significant impact on blood sugar levels.

• The apple cider vinegar and Dijon mustard in the dressing provide flavor without added sugars.

• The small amount of honey (if using) can help balance the acidity of the vinegar.

• It's a refreshing and crunchy side dish that can be enjoyed alongside grilled or roasted proteins.

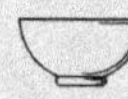 **Preparation Time : 15 min**

 **Total Time : 30 min - 1h**

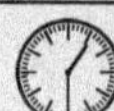 **Servings : 3-6**

Ingredients

• 4 cups shredded green cabbage
• 1 cup shredded red cabbage
• 1 medium carrot, peeled and grated
• 1 Granny Smith apple, cored and julienned
• 2 tbsp apple cider vinegar
• 1 tbsp olive oil
• 1 tsp Dijon mustard
• 1 tsp honey (optional)
• 1/4 tsp salt
• 1/8 tsp black pepper
• 2 tbsp chopped fresh parsley (optional)

Instructions

1. In a large salad bowl, combine the baby arugula, roasted and sliced beets, crumbled goat cheese, and toasted walnuts or pecans.

2. In a small bowl, whisk together the balsamic vinegar, olive oil, Dijon mustard, honey (if using), salt, and black pepper to make the dressing.

3. Drizzle the dressing over the salad and toss gently to coat the ingredients evenly.

4. Serve the arugula salad with beets and goat cheese immediately.

This salad is a great option for men managing type 2 diabetes for several reasons:

• Arugula is a leafy green that is low in carbs and high in vitamins and antioxidants.

• Beets are a root vegetable that are low in carbs and high in fiber, vitamins, and minerals.

• Goat cheese provides a creamy texture and a source of protein without a significant amount of carbs.

• The healthy fats from the olive oil and nuts can help improve insulin sensitivity.

• The small amount of honey (if using) provides a touch of sweetness without a major impact on blood sugar levels.

• The balsamic vinegar and Dijon mustard in the dressing add flavor without added sugars.

Enjoy this delicious arugula salad with beets and goat cheese!

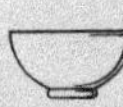 **Preparation Time : 15 min**

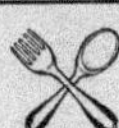 **Total Time : 30 min - 1h**

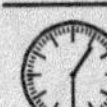 **Servings : 3-6**

Ingredients

• 5 oz baby arugula
• 2 medium beets, roasted, peeled, and sliced
• 2 oz crumbled goat cheese
• 2 tbsp toasted walnuts or pecans
• 2 tbsp balsamic vinegar
• 1 tbsp olive oil
• 1 tsp Dijon mustard
• 1 tsp honey (optional)
• 1/4 tsp salt
• 1/8 tsp black pepper

This salad is a refreshing and nutrient•dense option that can be enjoyed as a light main course or a side dish. It's a great way to incorporate more vegetables and healthy fats into a diabetes•friendly diet.

Instructions

1. In a small saucepan, combine the balsamic vinegar and honey (if using). Bring the mixture to a simmer over medium heat, stirring occasionally, until it has reduced by about half and thickened into a glaze, about 5•7 minutes. Remove from heat and let cool slightly.

2. Arrange the sliced mozzarella and tomatoes on a serving platter or individual plates. Scatter the fresh basil leaves over the top.

3. Drizzle the balsamic reduction over the salad, followed by the olive oil. Sprinkle with salt and black pepper.

4. Serve the caprese salad immediately.

This caprese salad is a great option for men managing type 2 diabetes for a few reasons:

• Tomatoes are low in carbs and high in antioxidants, which can help regulate blood sugar levels.

• Fresh mozzarella is a good source of protein and healthy fats.

• The balsamic reduction provides a sweet and tangy flavor without the need for added sugars.

• The small amount of olive oil helps with the absorption of fat•soluble vitamins from the tomatoes.

• The dish is light, refreshing, and can be easily incorporated into a balanced, diabetes•friendly diet.

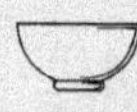 **Preparation Time : 15 min**

 **Total Time : 30 min - 1h**

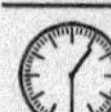 **Servings : 3-6**

Ingredients

• 8 oz fresh mozzarella cheese, sliced
• 2 medium tomatoes, sliced
• 1/4 cup fresh basil leaves
• 2 tbsp balsamic vinegar
• 1 tsp honey (optional)
• 1 tbsp olive oil
• 1/4 tsp salt
• 1/8 tsp black pepper

You can adjust the amount of balsamic reduction and honey to suit your taste preferences. Enjoy this delicious and nutritious caprese salad!

Instructions

1. Preheat oven to 400°F. Line a baking sheet with parchment paper.

2. In a large bowl, toss the zucchini, bell peppers, and red onion with the olive oil, oregano, garlic powder, salt, and pepper.

3. Spread the vegetables in a single layer on the prepared baking sheet. Roast for 20•25 minutes, stirring halfway, until vegetables are tender and lightly browned.

4. In a small bowl, whisk together the balsamic vinegar, Dijon mustard, and honey.

5. In a large salad bowl, combine the roasted vegetables and mixed greens. Drizzle the balsamic dressing over the top and toss gently to coat.

This salad is a great option for men with type 2 diabetes as it is high in fiber, low in carbs, and contains healthy fats from the olive oil. The roasted vegetables and balsamic dressing provide a flavorful and satisfying meal.

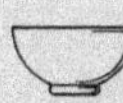 **Preparation Time : 15 min**

 **Total Time : 30 min - 1h**

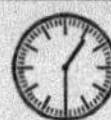 **Servings : 3-6**

Ingredients

- 1 medium zucchini, cut into 1•inch pieces
- 1 red bell pepper, cut into 1•inch pieces
- 1 yellow bell pepper, cut into 1•inch pieces
- 1 red onion, cut into 1•inch pieces
- 2 tbsp olive oil
- 1 tsp dried oregano
- 1/2 tsp garlic powder
- Salt and pepper to taste
- 5 oz mixed greens
- 2 tbsp balsamic vinegar
- 1 tbsp Dijon mustard
- 1 tbsp honey

87. Chickpea and Tomato Salad

Instructions

1. In a large bowl, combine the drained and rinsed chickpeas, halved tomatoes, and sliced red onion.

2. In a small bowl, whisk together the olive oil, red wine vinegar, Dijon mustard, and minced garlic. Season with salt and pepper.

3. Pour the dressing over the chickpea and tomato mixture and toss gently to coat.

4. Sprinkle the chopped fresh parsley over the top.

5. Refrigerate for at least 30 minutes before serving to allow the flavors to meld.

This salad is a great option for men with type 2 diabetes as it is high in fiber and protein from the chickpeas, and low in carbs. The healthy fats from the olive oil and the vinegar help to regulate blood sugar levels. Enjoy!

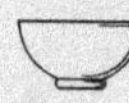 **Preparation Time : 15 min**

 **Total Time : 30 min - 1h**

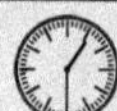 **Servings : 3-6**

Ingredients

- 1 (15 oz) can chickpeas, drained and rinsed
- 1 pint cherry or grape tomatoes, halved
- 1/2 red onion, thinly sliced
- 2 tbsp olive oil
- 2 tbsp red wine vinegar
- 1 tsp Dijon mustard
- 1 garlic clove, minced
- 1/4 cup chopped fresh parsley
- Salt and pepper to taste

Instructions

1. In a large bowl, combine the sliced cucumbers and red onion.

2. In a small bowl, whisk together the red wine vinegar, olive oil, Dijon mustard, and honey. Season with salt and pepper.

3. Pour the dressing over the cucumber and onion mixture and toss gently to coat.

4. Sprinkle with chopped fresh parsley if desired.

5. Refrigerate for at least 30 minutes before serving to allow the flavors to meld.

This salad is a great option for men with type 2 diabetes as it is low in carbs, high in fiber, and contains healthy fats from the olive oil. The vinegar and mustard also help to regulate blood sugar levels. Enjoy!

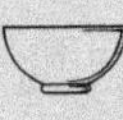 **Preparation Time : 15 min**

 **Total Time : 30 min - 1h**

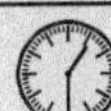 **Servings : 3-6**

Ingredients

- 2 medium cucumbers, sliced
- 1 small red onion, thinly sliced
- 2 tbsp red wine vinegar
- 1 tbsp olive oil
- 1 tsp Dijon mustard
- 1 tsp honey
- Salt and pepper to taste
- 2 tbsp chopped fresh parsley (optional)

Instructions

1. In a large bowl, combine the thinly sliced fennel, orange segments, and sliced red onion.

2. In a small bowl, whisk together the olive oil, lemon juice, Dijon mustard, and honey. Season with salt and pepper.

3. Pour the dressing over the fennel and orange mixture and toss gently to coat.

4. Sprinkle the chopped fresh parsley over the top.

5. Refrigerate for at least 30 minutes before serving to allow the flavors to meld.

This fennel and orange salad is a great option for men with type 2 diabetes for a few reasons:

1. Fennel is low in carbs and high in fiber, which can help regulate blood sugar levels.

2. Oranges are a good source of vitamin C and provide a sweet contrast to the licorice•like flavor of the fennel.

3. The olive oil, lemon juice, and Dijon mustard in the dressing provide healthy fats and help slow the absorption of sugars.

Enjoy this refreshing and flavorful salad!

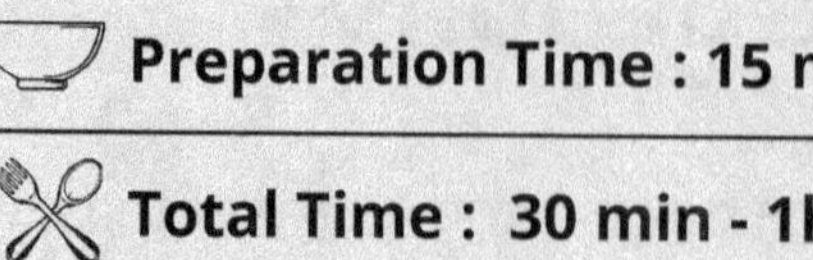

Ingredients

- 1 fennel bulb, thinly sliced
- 2 oranges, peeled and segmented
- 1/2 red onion, thinly sliced
- 2 tbsp olive oil
- 2 tbsp fresh lemon juice
- 1 tbsp Dijon mustard
- 1 tsp honey
- Salt and pepper to taste
- 2 tbsp chopped fresh parsley

Instructions

1. In a large bowl, combine the drained and rinsed chickpeas, diced cucumber, halved cherry tomatoes, sliced red onion, crumbled feta, and halved kalamata olives.

2. In a small bowl, whisk together the olive oil, red wine vinegar, dried oregano, and minced garlic. Season with salt and pepper.

3. Pour the dressing over the salad and toss gently to coat.

4. Sprinkle the chopped fresh parsley over the top.

5. Refrigerate for at least 30 minutes before serving to allow the flavors to meld.

This Greek salad is a great option for men with type 2 diabetes as it is high in fiber, protein, and healthy fats, while being low in carbs. The chickpeas, vegetables, and feta provide a satisfying and nutrient•dense meal. Enjoy!

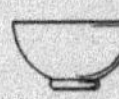 **Preparation Time : 15 min**

 **Total Time : 30 min - 1h**

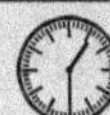 **Servings : 3-6**

Ingredients

- 1 (15 oz) can chickpeas, drained and rinsed
- 1 cucumber, diced
- 1 pint cherry tomatoes, halved
- 1/2 red onion, thinly sliced
- 1/2 cup crumbled feta cheese
- 1/4 cup kalamata olives, halved
- 2 tbsp olive oil
- 2 tbsp red wine vinegar
- 1 tsp dried oregano
- 1 garlic clove, minced
- Salt and pepper to taste
- 2 tbsp chopped fresh parsley

91. Baked Chicken with Herbs

Instructions

1. Preheat your oven to 400°F (200°C).

2. Pat the chicken breasts dry with paper towels and place them in a baking dish or on a rimmed baking sheet.

3. In a small bowl, mix together the olive oil, dried thyme, dried rosemary, garlic powder, and paprika. Season with salt and pepper.

4. Rub the herb mixture all over the chicken breasts, making sure to coat them evenly.

5. Bake the chicken in the preheated oven for 25•30 minutes, or until the internal temperature reaches 165°F (75°C).

6. Remove the chicken from the oven and let it rest for 5 minutes.

7. Sprinkle the chopped fresh parsley over the chicken, if using.

This baked chicken dish is a great option for men with type 2 diabetes for a few reasons:

• The chicken is a lean protein source, which is important for maintaining muscle mass and regulating blood sugar levels.

• The herbs and spices add flavor without the need for added sugars or sauces.

• Baking the chicken instead of frying it keeps the dish low in unhealthy fats.

Serve this chicken with a side of roasted vegetables or a fresh salad for a complete and diabetes•friendly meal.

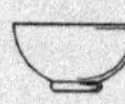 **Preparation Time : 15 min**

 **Total Time : 30 min - 1h**

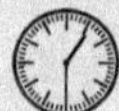 **Servings : 3-6**

Ingredients

• 4 boneless, skinless chicken breasts
• 2 tbsp olive oil
• 1 tsp dried thyme
• 1 tsp dried rosemary
• 1 tsp garlic powder
• 1/2 tsp paprika
• Salt and pepper to taste
• 2 tbsp chopped fresh parsley (optional)

Instructions

1. Preheat your grill or grill pan to medium•high heat.

2. In a shallow dish, combine the olive oil, lemon juice, lemon zest, oregano, and garlic powder. Season with salt and pepper.

3. Add the tilapia fillets to the dish and turn to coat both sides with the lemon•herb mixture.

4. Grill the tilapia for 3•4 minutes per side, or until it flakes easily with a fork.

5. Serve the grilled tilapia immediately, with lemon wedges on the side.

This grilled tilapia dish is an excellent choice for men with type 2 diabetes for several reasons:

• Tilapia is a lean, low•calorie source of protein that is high in omega•3 fatty acids, which can help improve insulin sensitivity.

• The lemon and herbs add flavor without the need for high•sugar sauces or marinades.

• Grilling the fish keeps it low in unhealthy fats, as opposed to frying.

Pair this grilled tilapia with a side of roasted vegetables or a fresh salad for a complete, diabetes•friendly meal. Enjoy!

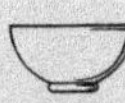 **Preparation Time : 15 min**

 **Total Time : 30 min - 1h**

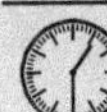 **Servings : 3-6**

Ingredients

• 4 tilapia fillets (about 1 lb total)
• 2 tbsp olive oil
• 2 tbsp fresh lemon juice
• 1 tsp grated lemon zest
• 1 tsp dried oregano
• 1/2 tsp garlic powder
• Salt and pepper to taste
• Lemon wedges for serving

Instructions

1. Preheat your oven to 400°F (200°C).

2. In a small bowl, mix together the olive oil, dried thyme, garlic powder, salt, and pepper. Rub this mixture all over the pork tenderloin.

3. Place the pork tenderloin in a baking dish and roast in the preheated oven for 25•30 minutes, or until the internal temperature reaches 145°F (63°C).

4. While the pork is roasting, prepare the apple sauce. In a saucepan, combine the diced apples, apple cider, lemon juice, and cinnamon. Bring the mixture to a simmer over medium heat.

5. Reduce the heat to low and let the apple sauce simmer for 10•15 minutes, stirring occasionally, until the apples are soft and the sauce has thickened.

6. Remove the pork tenderloin from the oven and let it rest for 5 minutes before slicing.

7. Serve the sliced pork tenderloin with the warm apple sauce on the side.

This pork tenderloin dish is a great option for men with type 2 diabetes for a few reasons:

• Pork tenderloin is a lean protein source that is low in fat and carbs.

• The apple sauce provides a sweet and tangy complement to the pork without the need for added sugars.

• The dish is baked, not fried, keeping it low in unhealthy fats.

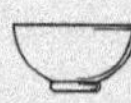 **Preparation Time : 15 min**

 **Total Time : 30 min - 1h**

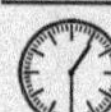 **Servings : 3-6**

Ingredients

• 1 lb pork tenderloin
• 1 tbsp olive oil
• 1 tsp dried thyme
• 1/2 tsp garlic powder
• Salt and pepper to taste
• 2 medium apples, peeled, cored, and diced
• 1/4 cup unsweetened apple cider
• 1 tbsp lemon juice
• 1 tsp ground cinnamon

Instructions

1. In a medium bowl, combine the sliced beef, soy sauce, rice vinegar, sesame oil, ginger, and garlic. Toss to coat and let marinate for 15 minutes.

2. Heat the olive oil in a large skillet or wok over high heat. Add the marinated beef and stir•fry for 2•3 minutes until browned.

3. Add the sliced bell pepper, broccoli, mushrooms, and snow peas. Stir•fry for 3•4 minutes until the vegetables are tender•crisp.

4. Remove from heat and stir in the sliced green onions. Season with salt and pepper to taste.

5. Serve immediately, over cauliflower rice or steamed brown rice if desired.

This beef stir•fry is a great option for men with type 2 diabetes as it is high in protein, low in carbs, and packed with fiber•rich vegetables. The soy sauce, vinegar, and ginger provide flavor without added sugar. Enjoy!

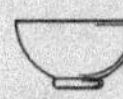 **Preparation Time : 15 min**

 **Total Time : 30 min - 1h**

 **Servings : 3-6**

Ingredients

- 1 lb lean beef sirloin, thinly sliced
- 2 tbsp low•sodium soy sauce
- 1 tbsp rice vinegar
- 1 tsp sesame oil
- 1 tsp grated ginger
- 2 cloves garlic, minced
- 2 tbsp olive oil
- 1 red bell pepper, sliced
- 1 cup broccoli florets
- 1 cup sliced mushrooms
- 1 cup snow peas
- 2 green onions, sliced
- Salt and pepper to taste

Instructions

1. Preheat your oven to 400°F (200°C).

2. Place the spaghetti squash halves cut•side up on a baking sheet. Drizzle the squash with 1 tbsp of the olive oil and season with salt and pepper.

3. Roast the spaghetti squash in the preheated oven for 40•50 minutes, or until the flesh is tender and can be easily shredded with a fork.

4. Remove the spaghetti squash from the oven and let it cool slightly. Using a fork, gently shred the flesh of the squash, creating long, spaghetti•like strands.

5. In a saucepan, heat the remaining 1 tbsp of olive oil over medium heat. Add the marinara sauce and heat through, stirring occasionally.

6. Divide the spaghetti squash strands among plates or bowls. Top each serving with the warm marinara sauce.

7. If desired, sprinkle the spaghetti squash and sauce with grated Parmesan cheese and chopped fresh basil leaves.

This spaghetti squash dish is a great low•carb alternative to traditional pasta. The spaghetti squash provides a similar texture and shape to pasta, but with fewer carbs and more fiber and nutrients.

Enjoy this delicious and healthy spaghetti squash dish!

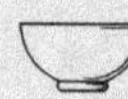 **Preparation Time : 15 min**

 **Total Time : 30 min - 1h**

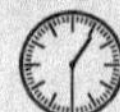 **Servings : 3-6**

Ingredients

• 1 medium spaghetti squash, halved lengthwise and seeds removed
• 2 tbsp olive oil
• 1 jar (24 oz) low•sodium marinara sauce
• 1/4 cup grated Parmesan cheese (optional)
• Fresh basil leaves, chopped (optional)

Some key benefits of this dish:

• Spaghetti squash is low in carbs and calories, making it a good option for those watching their blood sugar levels or trying to maintain a healthy weight.

• The marinara sauce provides a flavorful and nutrient•rich topping without the need for high•calorie or sugary sauces.

• The dish is gluten•free and can be easily adapted to be vegetarian or vegan by omitting the Parmesan cheese.

Instructions

1. Preheat your oven to 400°F (200°C). Line a baking sheet with parchment paper.

2. In a medium bowl, whisk together the soy sauce, rice vinegar, sesame oil, honey, grated ginger, and minced garlic.

3. Add the tofu cubes to the bowl and gently toss to coat them evenly with the soy sauce mixture.

4. Arrange the coated tofu cubes in a single layer on the prepared baking sheet.

5. Bake the tofu for 20•25 minutes, flipping the cubes halfway through, until they are golden brown and crispy.

6. Remove the baked tofu from the oven and sprinkle with sesame seeds and chopped green onions, if desired.

7. Serve the baked tofu warm, either on its own or over a bed of steamed rice or roasted vegetables.

This baked tofu dish is a great option for a healthy and flavorful meal. The soy sauce, ginger, and garlic provide a delicious Asian•inspired taste, while the baking method keeps the dish low in fat.

Enjoy this tasty and nutritious Baked Tofu with Soy Sauce!

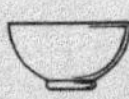 **Preparation Time : 15 min**

 **Total Time : 30 min - 1h**

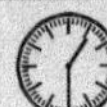 **Servings : 3-6**

Ingredients

• 1 block (14 oz) extra•firm tofu, drained and cut into 1•inch cubes
• 2 tbsp low•sodium soy sauce
• 1 tbsp rice vinegar
• 1 tsp sesame oil
• 1 tsp honey
• 1 tsp grated ginger
• 1 clove garlic, minced
• 1 tbsp sesame seeds (optional)
• 2 tbsp chopped green onions (optional)

Some key benefits of this recipe:

• Tofu is a great source of plant•based protein, making it a good option for vegetarians and vegans.

• The dish is low in carbs and calories, making it a suitable choice for those managing their blood sugar levels or trying to maintain a healthy weight.

• The baking method avoids the need for frying, which can add unhealthy fats to the dish.

Instructions

1. In a shallow dish, combine the olive oil, chopped rosemary, minced garlic, and lemon zest. Season the lamb chops with salt and pepper, then add them to the dish and turn to coat both sides.

2. Preheat your grill or grill pan to medium·high heat.

3. Grill the lamb chops for 3·4 minutes per side, or until they reach your desired level of doneness. The internal temperature should reach 145°F (63°C) for medium·rare, or 160°F (71°C) for medium.

4. Transfer the grilled lamb chops to a plate and let them rest for 5 minutes before serving.

This grilled lamb chop recipe is a delicious and flavorful option. The rosemary, garlic, and lemon zest provide a wonderful aroma and taste, while the grilling method keeps the dish lean and healthy.

Some key benefits of this dish:

• Lamb is a great source of protein, iron, and other essential nutrients.

• The rosemary and garlic add flavor without the need for high·calorie sauces or marinades.

• Grilling the lamb chops keeps the dish low in unhealthy fats, as opposed to frying.

• The dish is relatively low in carbs, making it a good option for those watching their blood sugar levels.

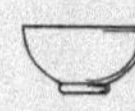 **Preparation Time : 15 min**

 **Total Time : 30 min - 1h**

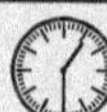 **Servings : 3-6**

Ingredients

• 8 lamb chops (about 1·1.5 lbs)
• 2 tbsp olive oil
• 2 tbsp fresh rosemary, chopped
• 2 cloves garlic, minced
• 1 tsp lemon zest
• Salt and pepper to taste

98. Chicken Fajitas with Bell Peppers

Instructions

1. In a large bowl, combine the sliced chicken, bell peppers, and onion. Drizzle with the olive oil and sprinkle with the chili powder, cumin, garlic powder, smoked paprika, salt, and pepper. Toss to coat the ingredients evenly.

2. Heat a large skillet or grill pan over medium•high heat. Add the chicken and vegetable mixture and cook, stirring occasionally, for 8•10 minutes or until the chicken is cooked through and the vegetables are tender•crisp.

3. Warm the whole wheat tortillas or lettuce wraps according to package instructions.

4. To serve, divide the chicken and vegetable mixture evenly among the tortillas or lettuce wraps. Top with your desired toppings, such as avocado, salsa, plain Greek yogurt, and/or shredded cheese.

This chicken fajita dish is a great option for a healthy and flavorful meal. The combination of lean protein, fresh vegetables, and whole grain tortillas or lettuce wraps makes it a nutritious choice.

Some key benefits of this recipe:

• The chicken and vegetables provide a good source of lean protein and fiber to help keep you feeling full and satisfied.

• The spices add flavor without the need for high•calorie sauces or marinades.

• Using whole wheat tortillas or lettuce wraps instead of traditional flour tortillas helps keep the carb content lower.

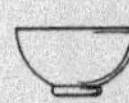 **Preparation Time : 15 min**

 **Total Time : 30 min - 1h**

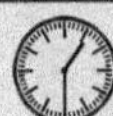 **Servings : 3-6**

Ingredients

• 1 lb boneless, skinless chicken breasts, sliced into thin strips
• 2 bell peppers (any color), sliced into thin strips
• 1 onion, sliced into thin strips
• 2 tbsp olive oil
• 2 tsp chili powder
• 1 tsp cumin
• 1 tsp garlic powder
• 1/2 tsp smoked paprika
• Salt and pepper to taste
• 8 small whole wheat tortillas or lettuce wraps
• Toppings (optional): avocado, salsa, plain Greek yogurt, shredded cheese

Instructions

1. Preheat your oven to 400°F (200°C). Line a baking sheet with parchment paper.

2. Gently clean the portobello mushroom caps with a damp paper towel. Remove and chop the stems.

3. In a skillet, heat the olive oil over medium heat. Add the chopped mushroom stems, diced onion, and minced garlic. Sauté for 3•4 minutes until the onion is translucent.

4. Add the chopped spinach to the skillet and cook for another 2•3 minutes, until the spinach is wilted.

5. Remove the skillet from heat and stir in the crumbled feta cheese, grated Parmesan cheese, and dried oregano. Season with salt and pepper to taste.

6. Arrange the portobello mushroom caps, gill•side up, on the prepared baking sheet. Spoon the spinach and cheese mixture evenly into the mushroom caps.

7. Bake the stuffed portobello mushrooms in the preheated oven for 15•20 minutes, or until the mushrooms are tender and the filling is hot and bubbly.

8. Serve the stuffed portobello mushrooms warm, garnished with additional Parmesan cheese or fresh herbs if desired.

These Stuffed Portobello Mushrooms make a delicious and nutritious vegetarian main dish or side. The combination of the meaty mushroom caps, nutrient•rich spinach, and flavorful cheeses creates a satisfying and diabetes•friendly meal.

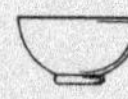 **Preparation Time : 15 min**

 **Total Time : 30 min - 1h**

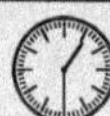 **Servings : 3-6**

Ingredients

• 4 large portobello mushroom caps, stems removed and chopped
• 1 tbsp olive oil
• 1/2 cup diced onion
• 2 cloves garlic, minced
• 1 cup baby spinach, chopped
• 1/2 cup crumbled feta cheese
• 2 tbsp grated Parmesan cheese
• 1 tsp dried oregano
• Salt and pepper to taste

Some key benefits of this recipe:

• Portobello mushrooms are low in carbs and calories, making them a great option for those managing their blood sugar levels.

• The spinach and feta provide a good source of fiber, vitamins, and minerals.

• The dish is baked, not fried, keeping it low in unhealthy fats.

• It's easily customizable with different vegetable or cheese fillings to suit your preferences.

Instructions

1. In a large bowl, combine the cooked shrimp, diced avocados, halved cherry tomatoes, and thinly sliced red onion.

2. In a small bowl, whisk together the olive oil, lime juice, and Dijon mustard. Season with salt and pepper.

3. Pour the dressing over the shrimp and avocado mixture and toss gently to coat.

4. Sprinkle the chopped fresh cilantro over the top.

5. Refrigerate for at least 30 minutes before serving to allow the flavors to meld.

This Shrimp and Avocado Salad is a great option for a light and refreshing meal. The combination of protein•rich shrimp, healthy fats from the avocado, and fresh vegetables makes it a nutritious and satisfying choice.

Some key benefits of this salad:

• High in protein and healthy fats to help keep you feeling full and satisfied.

• Low in carbs, making it a good option for those watching their blood sugar levels.

• The fresh lime juice and Dijon mustard dressing adds flavor without the need for high•calorie or sugary dressings.

• The avocado provides creaminess and additional nutrients like fiber, vitamins, and minerals.

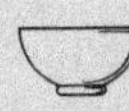 **Preparation Time : 15 min**

 **Total Time : 30 min - 1h**

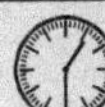 **Servings : 3-6**

Ingredients

• 1 lb cooked shrimp, peeled and deveined
• 2 avocados, diced
• 1 cup cherry tomatoes, halved
• 1/2 red onion, thinly sliced
• 2 tbsp fresh cilantro, chopped
• 2 tbsp olive oil
• 2 tbsp lime juice
• 1 tsp Dijon mustard
• Salt and pepper to taste

Instructions

1. Press the tofu for 15•30 minutes to remove excess moisture. Cut into 1•inch cubes.

2. Heat the vegetable oil in a large skillet or wok over medium•high heat. Add the tofu cubes and cook, turning occasionally, until lightly browned on all sides, about 5•7 minutes. Remove tofu from the pan and set aside.

3. Add the onion to the pan and cook for 2•3 minutes until translucent. Add the garlic and cook for 1 minute more.

4. Add the bell pepper, broccoli, mushrooms, and snow peas. Stir•fry for 4•5 minutes until the vegetables are tender•crisp.

5. Return the tofu to the pan. Add the soy sauce, rice vinegar, and sesame oil. Toss everything together and cook for 2•3 minutes more.

6. Season with salt and pepper to taste.

7. Serve the vegetable stir•fry immediately over steamed rice.

Enjoy your healthy and flavorful vegetable and tofu stir•fry!

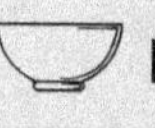 **Preparation Time : 15 min**

 **Total Time : 30 min - 1h**

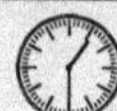 **Servings : 3-6**

Ingredients

- 1 block of firm or extra•firm tofu, cubed
- 2 tablespoons vegetable oil
- 1 onion, sliced
- 2 cloves garlic, minced
- 1 bell pepper, sliced
- 2 cups broccoli florets
- 1 cup sliced mushrooms
- 1 cup snow peas or snap peas
- 2 tablespoons soy sauce
- 1 tablespoon rice vinegar
- 1 teaspoon sesame oil
- Salt and pepper to taste
- Cooked rice, for serving

Instructions

1. Preheat your oven to 400°F (200°C). Line a baking sheet with parchment paper.

2. In a large bowl, toss the diced sweet potatoes with the olive oil, chili powder, cumin, salt, and pepper. Spread the seasoned sweet potatoes in a single layer on the prepared baking sheet.

3. Roast the sweet potatoes in the preheated oven for 20•25 minutes, or until they are tender and lightly browned, stirring halfway through.

4. In a medium bowl, combine the roasted sweet potatoes, drained and rinsed black beans, diced red onion, and chopped fresh cilantro. Stir to mix well.

5. Warm the whole wheat tortillas or lettuce wraps according to package instructions.

6. To assemble the tacos, spoon the black bean and sweet potato mixture into the center of each tortilla or lettuce wrap. Top with your desired toppings, such as diced avocado, salsa, plain Greek yogurt, and/or shredded cheese.

These Black Bean and Sweet Potato Tacos are a great option for men managing type 2 diabetes for several reasons:

• Sweet potatoes are a complex carbohydrate that is high in fiber and nutrients, helping to regulate blood sugar levels.
• Black beans provide protein and fiber, which can also help manage blood sugar.
• The whole wheat tortillas or lettuce wraps are a healthier alternative to traditional flour tortillas.
• The toppings can be customized to your preferences, allowing you to control the carb and calorie content.

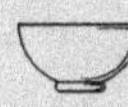 **Preparation Time : 15 min**

 **Total Time : 30 min - 1h**

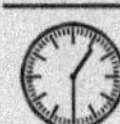 **Servings : 3-6**

Ingredients

• 2 medium sweet potatoes, peeled and diced
• 1 tbsp olive oil
• 1 tsp chili powder
• 1/2 tsp cumin
• Salt and pepper to taste
• 1 (15 oz) can black beans, drained and rinsed
• 1/2 cup diced red onion
• 2 tbsp chopped fresh cilantro
• 8•10 small whole wheat tortillas or lettuce wraps
• Toppings (optional): diced avocado, salsa, plain Greek yogurt, shredded cheese

Instructions

1. Preheat oven to 375°F. Place the bell pepper halves in a baking dish and set aside.

2. In a medium bowl, combine the cooked quinoa, black beans, diced tomatoes, onion, garlic, cumin, and chili powder. Mix well.

3. Spoon the quinoa mixture evenly into the bell pepper halves.

4. Sprinkle the crumbled feta cheese over the top of the stuffed peppers.

5. Bake for 25•30 minutes, until the peppers are tender and the filling is hot.

6. Serve immediately.

Why this is a great option for men with type 2 diabetes:

• Quinoa is a high•fiber, high•protein grain that is low in carbs and has a low glycemic index, making it a diabetes•friendly carb source.

• Black beans provide fiber, protein, and complex carbs without spiking blood sugar levels.

• Bell peppers are low in carbs and high in vitamins, minerals, and antioxidants.

• The dish is well•balanced with healthy fats from the feta cheese.

This stuffed pepper recipe is a nutritious, diabetes•friendly meal that is high in fiber, protein, and nutrients while being low in carbs and calories. It's a great option for men managing type 2 diabetes.

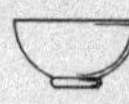 **Preparation Time : 15 min**

 **Total Time : 30 min - 1h**

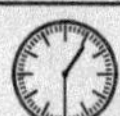 **Servings : 3-6**

Ingredients

• 4 bell peppers, halved lengthwise and seeds removed
• 1 cup cooked quinoa
• 1 (15 oz) can black beans, rinsed and drained
• 1 cup diced tomatoes
• 1/2 cup diced onion
• 2 cloves garlic, minced
• 1 tsp ground cumin
• 1 tsp chili powder
• 1/4 cup crumbled feta cheese
• Salt and pepper to taste

Instructions

1. In a large pot or Dutch oven, heat the olive oil over medium heat. Add the diced onion and sauté for 5 minutes until translucent.

2. Add the minced garlic, cumin, paprika, and cayenne (if using). Cook for 1 minute, stirring constantly, until fragrant.

3. Pour in the diced tomatoes, chickpeas, and broth. Bring the mixture to a simmer.

4. Reduce heat to medium•low and let the stew simmer for 15•20 minutes, until slightly thickened.

5. Stir in the chopped spinach and cook for 2•3 minutes more, until the spinach is wilted.

6. Season with salt and pepper to taste.

7. Serve the chickpea and spinach stew warm, garnished with chopped fresh parsley if desired.

Why this is a great option for men with type 2 diabetes:

• Chickpeas are a great source of fiber, protein, and complex carbs that won't spike blood sugar levels.
• Spinach is packed with vitamins, minerals, and antioxidants while being very low in carbs.
• The stew is low in calories and fat, but high in nutrients and fiber to help manage diabetes.
• The spices like cumin and paprika add flavor without adding sugar or carbs.

This hearty, diabetes•friendly stew is a nutritious and satisfying meal option for men managing type 2 diabetes.

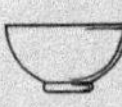 **Preparation Time : 15 min**

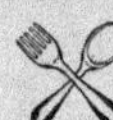 **Total Time : 30 min - 1h**

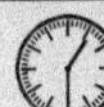 **Servings : 3-6**

Ingredients

• 2 tablespoons olive oil
• 1 onion, diced
• 3 cloves garlic, minced
• 2 teaspoons ground cumin
• 1 teaspoon paprika
• 1/4 teaspoon cayenne pepper (optional)
• 1 (15 oz) can diced tomatoes
• 1 (15 oz) can chickpeas, rinsed and drained
• 4 cups low•sodium vegetable or chicken broth
• 5 oz fresh spinach, chopped
• Salt and pepper to taste
• Chopped fresh parsley for garnish (optional)

Instructions

1. In a large bowl, combine the spiralized or julienned zucchini noodles with the basil pesto. Toss to coat the noodles evenly.

2. Transfer the zucchini noodles with pesto to a serving plate or bowl.

3. Sprinkle the toasted pine nuts and grated Parmesan cheese over the top.

4. Season with salt and pepper to taste.

That's it! This simple, no•cook dish is a great option for men managing type 2 diabetes for a few reasons:

1. Zucchini noodles are low in carbs and calories, making them a healthier alternative to traditional pasta.

2. Basil pesto is flavorful and contains healthy fats from the olive oil and pine nuts, without the added sugars found in many pasta sauces.

3. The dish is high in fiber, vitamins, and minerals from the zucchini and basil.

4. It's easy to prepare and can be enjoyed as a light main course or a side dish.

You can customize this recipe by using different types of pesto (e.g., arugula or kale pesto) or adding grilled chicken or shrimp for extra protein.

Enjoy this delicious and diabetes•friendly Zucchini Noodles with Pesto!

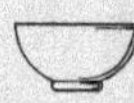 **Preparation Time : 15 min**

 **Total Time : 30 min - 1h**

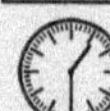 **Servings : 3-6**

Ingredients

• 3 medium zucchini, spiralized or julienned into noodles
• 1/2 cup basil pesto (store•bought or homemade)
• 2 tbsp toasted pine nuts
• 2 tbsp grated Parmesan cheese
• Salt and pepper to taste

Instructions

1. Preheat oven to 375°F. Grease a 9x13 baking dish.

2. In a medium saucepan, combine the lentils and vegetable broth. Bring to a boil, then reduce heat and simmer for 20•25 minutes until lentils are tender. Drain any excess liquid.

3. In a large skillet, heat the olive oil over medium heat. Add the onion and sauté for 5 minutes until translucent.

4. Add the mushrooms and cook for 5 more minutes. Stir in the garlic, thyme, rosemary, and tomato paste. Cook for 1 minute.

5. Add the cooked lentils and frozen peas to the skillet. Season with salt and pepper to taste.

6. Transfer the lentil•mushroom mixture to the prepared baking dish.

7. In a large pot, cover the potato chunks with water and bring to a boil. Reduce heat and simmer for 15•20 minutes until tender. Drain and return to the pot.

8. Mash the potatoes with the almond milk and butter until smooth. Spread the mashed potatoes over the lentil•mushroom filling. Top with Parmesan cheese if desired.

9. Bake for 30 minutes until the potatoes are lightly browned.

This hearty, diabetes•friendly shepherd's pie is packed with fiber, protein, and nutrients from the lentils, mushrooms, and potatoes. It's a comforting and satisfying meal option for men managing type 2 diabetes.

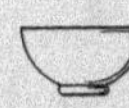 **Preparation Time : 15 min**

 **Total Time : 30 min - 1h**

 **Servings : 3-6**

Ingredients

Filling:
• 1 cup brown or green lentils, rinsed
• 4 cups low•sodium vegetable broth
• 1 tbsp olive oil
• 1 onion, diced
• 8 oz mushrooms, sliced
• 3 cloves garlic, minced
• 2 tsp dried thyme
• 1 tsp dried rosemary
• 1 tbsp tomato paste
• 1 cup frozen peas
• Salt and pepper to taste

Topping:
• 2 lbs russet or Yukon Gold potatoes, peeled and cut into 1•inch chunks
• 1/4 cup unsweetened almond milk
• 2 tbsp butter
• 1/4 cup grated Parmesan cheese (optional)

107. Eggplant and Tomato Bake

Instructions

1. Preheat oven to 375°F. Grease a 9x13 inch baking dish.

2. Arrange the eggplant slices in a single layer on a baking sheet. Brush both sides with 1 tablespoon of the olive oil. Bake for 15•20 minutes, flipping halfway, until eggplant is tender.

3. In a large skillet, heat the remaining 1 tablespoon of olive oil over medium heat. Add the diced onion and sauté for 5 minutes until translucent.

4. Add the minced garlic and cook for 1 minute more, until fragrant.

5. Pour in the can of diced tomatoes and stir in the oregano and basil. Season with salt and pepper to taste. Simmer for 10 minutes.

6. Arrange the roasted eggplant slices in the prepared baking dish. Pour the tomato sauce over the top, spreading it evenly.

7. Sprinkle the shredded mozzarella and grated Parmesan cheeses over the top.

8. Bake for 20•25 minutes, until the cheese is melted and lightly browned.

9. Let stand for 5 minutes before serving.

This eggplant and tomato bake is a delicious and healthy vegetarian dish. The roasted eggplant, tangy tomato sauce, and melty cheese make for a satisfying and flavorful meal. Enjoy!

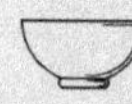 **Preparation Time : 15 min**

 **Total Time : 30 min - 1h**

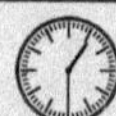 **Servings : 3-6**

Ingredients

- 1 large eggplant, cut into 1/2•inch thick slices
- 2 tablespoons olive oil, divided
- 1 onion, diced
- 3 cloves garlic, minced
- 1 (28 oz) can diced tomatoes
- 1 teaspoon dried oregano
- 1/2 teaspoon dried basil
- Salt and pepper to taste
- 1 cup shredded mozzarella cheese
- 1/4 cup grated Parmesan cheese

Instructions

1. Preheat oven to 400°F. Line a baking sheet with parchment paper.

2. In a large bowl, toss the cauliflower florets with the olive oil, chili powder, cumin, garlic powder, salt, and pepper until evenly coated.

3. Spread the seasoned cauliflower in a single layer on the prepared baking sheet.

4. Roast for 20•25 minutes, stirring halfway, until the cauliflower is tender and lightly browned.

5. Warm the tortillas according to package instructions.

6. To assemble the tacos, place some of the roasted cauliflower in each tortilla. Top with shredded cabbage, avocado slices, crumbled feta, and chopped cilantro.

7. Serve the cauliflower tacos immediately with lime wedges on the side.

These cauliflower tacos make a delicious and nutritious vegetarian/vegan•friendly meal. The roasted cauliflower has a great texture and flavor that pairs perfectly with the fresh toppings. Feel free to customize the toppings to your liking. Enjoy!

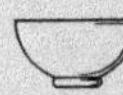 **Preparation Time : 15 min**

 **Total Time : 30 min - 1h**

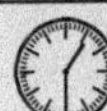 **Servings : 3-6**

Ingredients

- 1 head of cauliflower, cut into florets
- 2 tablespoons olive oil
- 1 teaspoon chili powder
- 1 teaspoon cumin
- 1/2 teaspoon garlic powder
- Salt and pepper to taste
- 8•10 small corn or flour tortillas
- 1 cup shredded cabbage or lettuce
- 1 avocado, sliced
- 1/4 cup crumbled feta or queso fresco
- Chopped cilantro for garnish
- Lime wedges for serving

109. Vegetable Paella

Instructions

1. In a large, oven•safe skillet or paella pan, heat the olive oil over medium heat. Add the diced onion and sauté for 3•4 minutes until translucent.

2. Add the minced garlic, diced bell pepper, sliced mushrooms, frozen peas, and diced zucchini. Sauté for another 5 minutes, stirring occasionally.

3. Stir in the uncooked brown rice, vegetable broth, smoked paprika, and saffron (if using). Season with salt and pepper.

4. Bring the mixture to a boil, then reduce heat to low, cover, and simmer for 25•30 minutes, or until the rice is tender and has absorbed most of the liquid.

5. Remove the lid and transfer the paella to the oven. Bake at 400°F (200°C) for 10•15 minutes, or until the rice is lightly browned on top.

6. Remove the paella from the oven and sprinkle with the chopped fresh parsley.

7. Serve the vegetable paella immediately, while hot.

This vegetable paella is a great option for men with type 2 diabetes for several reasons:

• It's high in fiber, vitamins, and minerals from the variety of vegetables.
• The brown rice provides complex carbs, which are digested more slowly than refined grains.
• The dish is low in calories and fat, as it's not made with any meat or seafood.

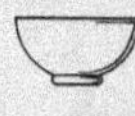
Preparation Time : 15 min

Total Time : 30 min - 1h

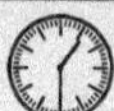
Servings : 3-6

Ingredients

• 1 tbsp olive oil
• 1 onion, diced
• 3 cloves garlic, minced
• 1 red bell pepper, diced
• 1 cup sliced mushrooms
• 1 cup frozen peas
• 1 cup diced zucchini
• 1 cup uncooked short•grain brown rice
• 2 cups low•sodium vegetable broth
• 1 tsp smoked paprika
• 1/2 tsp saffron threads (optional)
• Salt and pepper to taste
• 2 tbsp chopped fresh parsley

Instructions

1. Preheat oven to 400°F. Toss the cubed butternut squash with 1 tbsp of the olive oil on a baking sheet. Roast for 20•25 minutes, until tender and lightly browned. Set aside.

2. In a large saucepan, heat the remaining 1 tbsp olive oil over medium heat. Add the diced onion and sauté for 5 minutes until translucent.

3. Add the minced garlic and Arborio rice. Cook for 2•3 minutes, stirring frequently, until the rice is lightly toasted.

4. Pour in the white wine and cook, stirring constantly, until the wine is absorbed, about 2 minutes.

5. Ladle in 1/2 cup of the hot broth and cook, stirring frequently, until the liquid is absorbed. Continue this process, adding 1/2 cup of broth at a time, until the rice is tender and creamy, about 20•25 minutes total.

6. Stir in the roasted butternut squash, Parmesan cheese, and chopped sage. Season with salt and pepper to taste.

7. Serve the butternut squash risotto immediately.

This creamy, flavorful risotto makes a wonderful main dish or side for men managing type 2 diabetes.

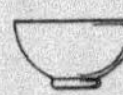 **Preparation Time : 15 min**

 **Total Time : 30 min - 1h**

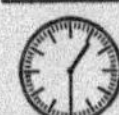 **Servings : 3-6**

Ingredients

• 1 small butternut squash, peeled, seeded, and cubed (about 3 cups)
• 2 tbsp olive oil, divided
• 1 onion, diced
• 2 cloves garlic, minced
• 1 cup Arborio rice
• 1/2 cup dry white wine
• 4 cups low•sodium chicken or vegetable broth, heated
• 1/4 cup grated Parmesan cheese
• 2 tbsp chopped fresh sage
• Salt and pepper to taste

Why this is a great option for men with type 2 diabetes:

• Butternut squash is low in carbs and high in fiber, vitamins, and antioxidants.
• Arborio rice has a lower glycemic index than regular white rice.
• The dish is balanced with a moderate amount of healthy fats from the olive oil and Parmesan.
• It's a satisfying, diabetes•friendly meal that is high in nutrients.

Instructions

1. Preheat oven to 325°F. Remove the giblets and neck from the turkey cavity and discard or save for another use.

2. Place the onion, carrots, celery, thyme, and rosemary in the turkey cavity. Rub the outside of the turkey all over with the softened butter. Season with 1 tsp salt and 1/2 tsp pepper.

3. Place the turkey, breast-side up, on a rack in a large roasting pan. Pour the broth into the bottom of the pan.

4. Roast the turkey for 2.5-3 hours, basting every 30 minutes, until a meat thermometer inserted into the thickest part of the thigh reads 165°F.

5. Meanwhile, toss the potato chunks and Brussels sprouts with the olive oil, 1 tsp salt, and 1/2 tsp pepper on a large baking sheet.

6. During the last 1 hour of turkey roasting, add the vegetable tray to the oven. Roast the vegetables until tender and lightly browned, about 45-60 minutes.

7. Transfer the turkey to a cutting board and let rest for 20-30 minutes before carving.

8. Serve the roast turkey with the roasted vegetables on the side.

This classic roast turkey with a medley of roasted vegetables makes for a delicious and satisfying holiday meal. Enjoy!

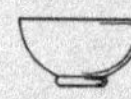 **Preparation Time : 15 min**

 **Total Time : 30 min - 1h**

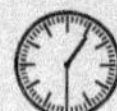 **Servings : 3-6**

Ingredients

• 1 (12-14 lb) whole turkey, thawed if frozen
• 1 onion, quartered
• 3 carrots, peeled and cut into 2-inch pieces
• 3 celery stalks, cut into 2-inch pieces
• 4 sprigs fresh thyme
• 4 sprigs fresh rosemary
• 1/2 cup unsalted butter, softened
• 1 tsp salt
• 1/2 tsp black pepper
• 4 cups low-sodium chicken or turkey broth

For the Vegetables:
• 3 lbs Yukon Gold potatoes, peeled and cut into 1-inch chunks
• 2 lbs Brussels sprouts, trimmed and halved
• 2 tbsp olive oil
• 1 tsp salt
• 1/2 tsp black pepper

Instructions

1. Make the mango salsa: In a medium bowl, combine the diced mango, red onion, jalapeño, cilantro, lime juice, and 1/4 teaspoon salt. Stir to mix well and set aside.

2. Prepare the swordfish: Pat the swordfish steaks dry with paper towels. Brush both sides with the olive oil and season with the chili powder, garlic powder, salt, and pepper.

3. Preheat a grill or grill pan to medium•high heat.

4. Grill the swordfish for 4•5 minutes per side, until cooked through and opaque in the center.

5. Transfer the grilled swordfish to plates and top each steak with a generous amount of the mango salsa.

6. Serve the swordfish immediately, with any extra salsa on the side.

The sweet and spicy mango salsa is the perfect complement to the grilled swordfish. This healthy and flavorful dish is sure to impress. Enjoy!

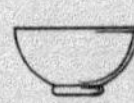 **Preparation Time : 15 min**

 **Total Time : 30 min - 1h**

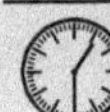 **Servings : 3-6**

Ingredients

For the Mango Salsa:
• 1 ripe mango, diced
• 1/2 red onion, finely chopped
• 1 jalapeño, seeded and finely chopped
• 1/4 cup chopped fresh cilantro
• 2 tablespoons lime juice
• 1/4 teaspoon salt

For the Swordfish:
• 4 (6 oz) swordfish steaks
• 2 tablespoons olive oil
• 1 teaspoon chili powder
• 1/2 teaspoon garlic powder
• 1/2 teaspoon salt
• 1/4 teaspoon black pepper

Instructions

1. Preheat oven to 400°F. Place the acorn squash halves cut•side up on a baking sheet. Brush the insides with 1 tbsp of the olive oil and season with salt and pepper.

2. Roast the squash for 30•40 minutes, until tender when pierced with a fork.

3. Meanwhile, in a large skillet, cook the Italian sausage over medium heat, breaking it up with a wooden spoon, until browned, about 5•7 minutes. Drain any excess fat.

4. Add the remaining 1 tbsp olive oil to the skillet along with the diced onion. Sauté for 5 minutes until the onion is translucent.

5. Stir in the minced garlic and cook for 1 minute more.

6. Remove the skillet from heat and stir in the cooked quinoa, chopped spinach, mozzarella, Parmesan, and oregano. Season with salt and pepper.

7. Scoop the sausage•quinoa mixture into the roasted acorn squash halves, dividing it evenly.

8. Return the stuffed squash to the oven and bake for 10•15 minutes, until the cheese is melted.

9. Serve the stuffed acorn squash warm.

This hearty, vegetable•based dish is a delicious and nutritious meal. The sweet roasted squash pairs perfectly with the savory sausage and quinoa stuffing. Enjoy!

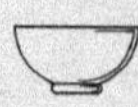 **Preparation Time : 15 min**

 **Total Time : 30 min - 1h**

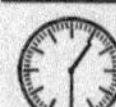 **Servings : 3-6**

Ingredients

- 2 acorn squash, halved lengthwise and seeds removed
- 2 tbsp olive oil, divided
- 1 lb Italian sausage, casings removed
- 1 onion, diced
- 3 cloves garlic, minced
- 1 cup cooked quinoa
- 1 cup baby spinach, chopped
- 1/2 cup shredded mozzarella cheese
- 1/4 cup grated Parmesan cheese
- 1 tsp dried oregano
- Salt and pepper to taste

Instructions

1. Preheat oven to 400°F.

2. Pat the beef tenderloin dry and rub all over with the olive oil, salt, and pepper.

3. Place the tenderloin on a rimmed baking sheet. Roast for 30•40 minutes, until it reaches your desired doneness (125°F for medium•rare, 130•135°F for medium).

4. Transfer the tenderloin to a cutting board and let rest for 10 minutes before slicing.

5. While the tenderloin is resting, make the red wine sauce. In a small saucepan, combine the red wine and beef broth. Bring to a simmer over medium heat and cook until reduced by half, about 10 minutes.

6. Reduce heat to low and whisk in the butter, shallot, Dijon, thyme, salt, and pepper. Cook for 2•3 minutes, until slightly thickened.

7. Slice the beef tenderloin and serve immediately, drizzled with the red wine sauce.

This elegant beef tenderloin with a rich red wine sauce makes a wonderful main dish for men managing type 2 diabetes.

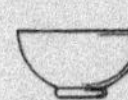 **Preparation Time : 15 min**

 **Total Time : 30 min - 1h**

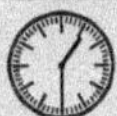 **Servings : 3-6**

Ingredients

• 2 lbs beef tenderloin, trimmed
• 2 tbsp olive oil
• 1 tsp salt
• 1/2 tsp black pepper

For the Red Wine Sauce:
• 1 cup dry red wine
• 1 cup low•sodium beef broth
• 2 tbsp unsalted butter
• 2 tbsp finely chopped shallot
• 2 tsp Dijon mustard
• 1 tsp fresh thyme leaves
• 1/4 tsp salt
• 1/8 tsp black pepper

Why this is a great option for men with type 2 diabetes:

• Beef tenderloin is a lean, high•protein cut of meat that is low in carbs.
• The red wine sauce provides flavor without adding a lot of sugar or carbs.
• The dish is balanced with healthy fats from the olive oil and butter.
• It's a satisfying, diabetes•friendly meal that is high in protein and nutrients.

Instructions

1. Preheat oven to 325°F.

2. Season the lamb shanks all over with salt and pepper.

3. In a large Dutch oven or heavy•bottomed pot, heat the olive oil over medium•high heat. Working in batches if needed, brown the lamb shanks on all sides, about 3•4 minutes per side. Transfer to a plate.

4. Reduce heat to medium and add the diced onion to the pot. Cook for 5 minutes until translucent. Add the garlic and cook for 1 minute more.

5. Pour in the red wine and use a wooden spoon to scrape up any browned bits from the bottom of the pot. Let the wine simmer for 2•3 minutes.

6. Return the browned lamb shanks to the pot and pour in the beef or chicken broth. Add the rosemary sprigs and bay leaves.

7. Cover the pot and transfer to the preheated oven. Braise the lamb shanks for 2•2.5 hours, until the meat is very tender and falling off the bone.

8. Meanwhile, make the mint sauce by combining all the sauce ingredients in a small bowl. Stir well and set aside.

9. Remove the pot from the oven. Transfer the cooked lamb shanks to a serving platter.

10. Serve the lamb shanks warm, drizzled with the mint sauce.

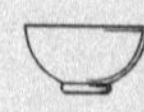 **Preparation Time : 15 min**

 **Total Time : 30 min - 1h**

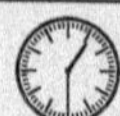 **Servings : 3-6**

Ingredients

For the Lamb Shanks:
• 4 lamb shanks
• 2 tbsp olive oil
• 1 onion, diced
• 3 cloves garlic, minced
• 1 cup dry red wine
• 2 cups low•sodium beef or chicken broth
• 2 sprigs fresh rosemary
• 2 bay leaves
• Salt and pepper to taste

For the Mint Sauce:
• 1 cup fresh mint leaves, finely chopped
• 2 tbsp red wine vinegar
• 1 tbsp honey
• 1 tsp Dijon mustard
• 1/4 tsp salt

Instructions

1. Preheat grill to medium·high heat.

2. Using kitchen shears, cut along the underside of each lobster tail, cutting all the way through the shell but leaving the meat intact.

3. In a small bowl, whisk together the olive oil, lemon juice, paprika, garlic powder, and cayenne (if using). Season with salt and pepper.

4. Brush the lobster tails all over with the seasoned oil mixture.

5. Grill the lobster tails, meat·side down, for 4·5 minutes. Flip and grill for another 4·5 minutes, until the meat is opaque and cooked through.

6. Transfer the grilled lobster tails to a serving platter. Serve immediately with lemon wedges.

Why this is a great option for men with type 2 diabetes:

• Lobster is an excellent source of lean protein that is low in carbs and calories.
• The simple seasoning of lemon, garlic, and paprika adds flavor without added sugars or unhealthy fats.
• Grilling the lobster tails requires no added oils or butter, keeping the dish low in fat.
• Lobster is rich in nutrients like selenium, zinc, and B vitamins that are important for diabetes management.

This elegant grilled lobster tail dish makes a delicious and diabetes·friendly main course. Pair it with a fresh salad or steamed vegetables for a complete, nutritious meal.

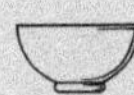 **Preparation Time : 15 min**

 **Total Time : 30 min - 1h**

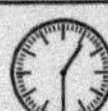 **Servings : 3-6**

Ingredients

• 4 (4·6 oz) lobster tails, thawed if frozen
• 2 tbsp olive oil
• 1 tbsp lemon juice
• 1 tsp paprika
• 1/2 tsp garlic powder
• 1/4 tsp cayenne pepper (optional)
• Salt and pepper to taste
• Lemon wedges for serving

Instructions

1. Preheat oven to 400°F. Line a large baking sheet with parchment paper.

2. In a small bowl, combine the minced garlic, chopped rosemary, olive oil, salt, and pepper. Mix well.

3. Place the Cornish hen halves skin•side up on the prepared baking sheet. Rub the garlic•rosemary mixture all over the hens, making sure to get it under the skin as well.

4. Roast the Cornish hens for 35•40 minutes, until the skin is crispy and the juices run clear when pierced with a fork. The internal temperature should reach 165°F.

5. Remove the hens from the oven and let rest for 5 minutes before serving.

6. Serve the Cornish hens warm, with lemon wedges on the side for squeezing over the top.

Tips:
• You can use whole Cornish hens instead of halves if preferred. Adjust the cooking time accordingly.
• For extra crispy skin, pat the hens very dry with paper towels before seasoning.
• Baste the hens with the pan juices halfway through cooking.
• Serve the Cornish hens with roasted vegetables or a fresh salad for a complete meal.

The combination of fragrant rosemary and garlic makes this Cornish hen dish incredibly flavorful. It's an elegant and easy•to•prepare main course that's perfect for a special occasion.

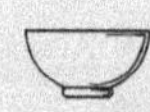 **Preparation Time : 15 min**

 **Total Time : 30 min - 1h**

 **Servings : 3-6**

Ingredients

• 2 Cornish hens, halved
• 4 cloves garlic, minced
• 2 tbsp fresh rosemary, chopped
• 2 tbsp olive oil
• 1 tsp salt
• 1/2 tsp black pepper
• 1 lemon, cut into wedges (for serving)

118. Stuffed Cabbage Rolls

Instructions

1. Bring a large pot of water to a boil. Using a paring knife, carefully cut out the core of the cabbage. Place the whole cabbage head in the boiling water and cook for 3•5 minutes, until the outer leaves are softened. Remove the cabbage and let cool slightly.

2. Carefully peel off the softened cabbage leaves, keeping them intact. You should get about 12•14 leaves.

3. In a large bowl, combine the ground beef/turkey, cooked rice, onion, garlic, egg, oregano, basil, salt, and pepper. Mix well.

4. Place about 1/4 cup of the meat mixture onto the center of each cabbage leaf. Fold the sides of the leaf over the filling, then roll up tightly.

5. Arrange the stuffed cabbage rolls seam•side down in a large baking dish or pot.

6. In a medium bowl, mix together the tomato sauce, diced tomatoes, and brown sugar (if using). Pour the sauce over the cabbage rolls.

7. Cover the dish and bake at 350°F for 60•75 minutes, until the cabbage is very tender and the filling is cooked through.

8. Serve the stuffed cabbage rolls warm, spooning extra sauce over the top.

These hearty, flavorful stuffed cabbage rolls make a delicious and comforting main dish. Enjoy!

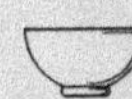 **Preparation Time : 15 min**

 **Total Time : 30 min - 1h**

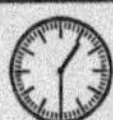 **Servings : 3-6**

Ingredients

- 1 medium head green cabbage
- 1 lb ground beef or ground turkey
- 1 cup cooked rice
- 1 onion, finely chopped
- 2 cloves garlic, minced
- 1 egg, beaten
- 1 tsp dried oregano
- 1 tsp dried basil
- 1/2 tsp salt
- 1/4 tsp black pepper
- 1 (15 oz) can tomato sauce
- 1 (15 oz) can diced tomatoes
- 1 tbsp brown sugar (optional)

Instructions

1. Preheat oven to 400°F. Line a baking sheet with parchment paper.

2. Pat the salmon fillet dry and season all over with salt and pepper.

3. In a skillet, heat the olive oil over medium·high heat. Sear the salmon on both sides until lightly browned, about 2·3 minutes per side. Remove from heat and let cool slightly.

4. In the same skillet, sauté the chopped mushrooms, shallot, and garlic until the mushrooms are tender and any liquid has evaporated, about 5·7 minutes. Deglaze the pan with the white wine and cook for 1 minute more. Stir in the heavy cream and season with salt and pepper.

5. On a lightly floured surface, roll out the puff pastry sheet to a rectangle large enough to fully wrap the salmon fillet.

6. Place the seared salmon fillet in the center of the pastry. Spoon the mushroom mixture over the top, spreading it to cover the salmon.

7. Fold the pastry over the salmon, pressing to seal the seams and edges. Place the wrapped salmon seam·side down on the prepared baking sheet.

8. Brush the top and sides of the pastry with the egg wash.

9. Bake for 25·30 minutes, until the pastry is golden brown.

10. Let the Salmon Wellington rest for 5·10 minutes before slicing and serving.

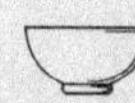 **Preparation Time : 15 min**

 **Total Time : 30 min - 1h**

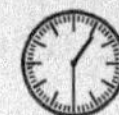 **Servings : 3-6**

Ingredients

- 1 lb salmon fillet, skin removed
- 1 tbsp olive oil
- 1 sheet frozen puff pastry, thawed
- 8 oz mushrooms, finely chopped
- 1 shallot, minced
- 2 cloves garlic, minced
- 2 tbsp dry white wine
- 2 tbsp heavy cream
- 1 egg, beaten with 1 tbsp water for egg wash
- Salt and pepper to taste

Instructions

1. Pat the scallops very dry with paper towels. Season them all over with salt and pepper.

2. Heat the olive oil in a large skillet over high heat. Working in batches if needed, add the scallops in a single layer and sear for 2•3 minutes per side, until a nice golden•brown crust forms.

3. Transfer the seared scallops to a plate and cover to keep warm.

4. Reduce the heat to medium and add the butter to the skillet. Cook, swirling the pan, until the butter is melted and starting to brown, about 2 minutes.

5. Remove the skillet from heat and stir in the lemon juice, parsley, and lemon zest. Season the lemon butter with salt and pepper to taste.

6. Spoon the warm lemon butter over the seared scallops and serve immediately.

Tips:
• Make sure the scallops are very dry before searing to get a nice caramelized crust.
• Don't overcrowd the pan when searing the scallops • work in batches if needed.
• Basting the scallops with the butter as they cook can help them develop more color.
• Serve the scallops with roasted vegetables, a fresh salad, or crusty bread to soak up the lemon butter.

This quick and elegant dish features perfectly seared scallops with a bright, flavorful lemon butter sauce. It's an impressive yet easy•to•prepare meal.

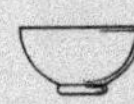 **Preparation Time : 15 min**

 **Total Time : 30 min - 1h**

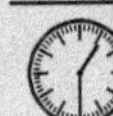 **Servings : 3-6**

Ingredients

• 1 lb sea scallops, patted dry
• 2 tbsp olive oil
• 3 tbsp unsalted butter
• 2 tbsp freshly squeezed lemon juice
• 1 tbsp chopped fresh parsley
• 1 tsp grated lemon zest
• Salt and pepper to taste

www.ingramcontent.com/pod-product-compliance
Lightning Source LLC
Chambersburg PA
CBHW081308250726
48662CB00008B/2449

9798332472947